# BRAINS LIKE OURS

# BRAINS LIKE OURS

A Smart Girl's Guide to Mood, Modern Life,
and the Science Behind Mental Health

TYLA BEE, CLS

Published by:
Redwood Publishing, LLC
Orange County, California
www.redwooddigitalpublishing.com

ISBN: 978-1-966333-34-0 hardcover)
ISBN: 978-1-966333-35-7 (paperback)
ISBN: 978-1-966333-26-5 (e-book)

Front cover design: Ink.Sharia
Full cover design: Kayode James O.
Interior design: JBookDesigns
Back cover author photograph: Tyla Bee

For speaking engagement inquiries or to buy books in bulk, contact the author directly at thetylabee@gmail.com

# CONTENTS

## PART 3: MOVE YOUR MIND—THE SCIENCE AND SOUL OF SWEAT

## PART 4: BECAUSE EVEN YOUR BRAIN NEEDS A GROUP CHAT



## PART 5: MIND OVER MATTER (AND MOOD): THE CASE FOR MINDFULNESS IN A CHAOTIC WORLD

**PART 6: DO SOMETHING USELESS: THE LIFE-SAVING MAGIC OF HOBBIES**

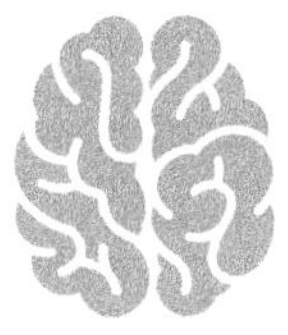



# CHAPTER 1

# THIS ISN'T A SELF-HELP BOOK; IT'S A SURVIVAL MANUAL

Welcome to the Work Hard, Die Hard Olympics, where burnout is a badge of honor and cortisol is the house wine. You don't win medals here, just migraines and performance anxiety.

I was staring at my dog while she ate breakfast like *Why is her life more regulated than mine?* If you're reading this, chances are you're somewhere between "I'm fine" and "Is it normal to break down in the bathroom at work?" You're probably the strong one. The responsible one. The one everyone leans on while you're quietly falling apart. And no matter how many planners you buy, supplements you try, or podcasts you listen to, you still feel like you're one step from catastrophically crumbling. I get it.

Has anyone else noticed that burnout is the baseline, and "trying your best" feels like screaming into a void? The pandemic may be technically over, but the aftermath is still showing up in our bodies and minds. We're still dealing with the emotional hangover of isolation, the nervous system dysregulation of too much bad news, and the quiet dread of trying to plan a future in an economy that feels like it was designed by Loki.

You start your day being jolted out of sleep by an alarm that feels more like a personal attack. You're immediately bombarded by emails, texts, to-dos, and the internal pressure to become a better version of yourself before 9 a.m. You try to get dressed without spiraling, then open Instagram just to "check one thing," and somehow end up comparing your sad eggs to the oat milk masterpiece someone has whipped up while hard launching their million-dollar lifestyle in pastel tones.

Your therapist raised her rates, your insurance doesn't cover anything useful, and the only doctor you can afford tells you your labs are "fine" while you sob alone in your car while eating dry granola.

Not to mention that your job is quietly bleeding you dry, and your hormones have decided to stage a protest via bloating, rage, and random chin hairs. And still, you're expected to "eat clean," "move your body," "practice gratitude," and "manifest abundance." Oh, and don't forget to recycle, support the locals, attend every birthday dinner, remember your cousin's baby's name, and stay hydrated. It's like trying to stay balanced on a tightrope while your hormones throw tomatoes at you.

We laugh about it online, but deep down, a lot of us are quietly suffering. You can't fix chronic overwhelm with lavender oil and discipline. You fix it by understanding the brain that's breaking under it, and I'm here to give you the tools I wish someone handed me before I lost two decades to anxiety and self-abandonment.

This book? It's not here to sell you a productivity hack or slap an affirmation over your panic. It's here because the system isn't working, your nervous system is exhausted, and your brain deserves better. And so do you. This book acknowledges that mental struggle doesn't show up the same way for everyone. Especially if you're a woman, neurodivergent, BIPOC, queer, or all of the above, the systems weren't made for you. And we're not here to gaslight that away.

Your nervous system doesn't speak English. It speaks physiology. Which is why this works when affirmations don't.

Here's your first win: When you inhale for four seconds and exhale for eight, your amygdala stops sounding the alarm faster than any affirmation or pep talk. Try it the next time you feel your pulse spike. You'll feel the drop within seconds.

Why does this work? When you lengthen your exhale, you're activating the parasympathetic branch of your autonomic nervous system. That sends an inhibitory signal through the vagus nerve, which lowers heart rate and dampens the amygdala's threat response. The longer exhale raises vagal tone, which tells your brain you're not in danger.

In other words, slower in, longer out equals a measurable shift in physiological arousal. It's basic neurophysiology doing more heavy lifting than any mantra ever could.

If you keep pushing through on fumes, your brain will adapt to that chaos. It will start treating stress as normal, rest as suspicious, and joy as an accident. You don't want that. No woman deserves to spend her life surviving herself.

This book is part survival guide, part science manual, and part love letter to anyone who's technically functioning but secretly dreams of getting a passport to the moon, forever. This isn't about escaping the chaos entirely; life is always going to be a little messy. Instead, it's about learning how we can thrive in the madness. It's about giving ourselves the important tools to feel human again without the overwhelm.

Before we get started, let me introduce my type-A self. I'm Tyla Bee, a clinical scientist who's had more panic attacks than I can name, faked injuries to leave a basic yoga class, doomscrolled through mental fog, and unknowingly found comfort in escapism and some other unhealthy habits. For years, I chased calm in all the wrong directions: too much work, too much noise, too many distractions. Each fix worked . . . until it didn't.

I've done the therapy roller coaster: the good, the bad, and the therapist who ghosted me (yes, that really happened). I've tried medications, and if they work for you, amazing! Personally? My brain responded by doing a full-blown frenzy, but we will talk about that in a bit. Not cute.

I was sixteen when someone finally gave my sadness a name. A psychologist looked at me and said "chronic depression." I didn't even know what depression was. I just knew I felt . . . heavy. Disconnected. Like my joy had an expiration date no one told me about.

Maybe it was a self-fulfilling prophecy. Maybe it was just my predetermined wiring. But the shadow never really left for a while. It showed up during the worst times: a hormonal dip, every winter, and honestly every life change. Sometimes it appeared for no reason at all, just because the sun rose that day. It was always in the background, but during moments of change—regardless of good or bad—my anxiety and depression would skyrocket, leaving me taxed and mentally drained. Every shift in my life, good or bad, felt like my brain had mistaken that growth for threat.

Change is the body's alarm clock; it wakes every cell in our bodies that thought they were safe. We don't just experience change logically; we *feel* it as anxiety or even depression. That's why we cling to routines, to sameness, because predictability feels better. The trick isn't to force comfort where there isn't any. It's to breathe long enough to let your brain learn that the new landscape isn't a battlefield. Hindsight is twenty-twenty.

When I was in my twenties I started my second go at therapy; it takes many, many times to get it right. If you know, you know. My parents were divorcing. My friend group diminished following a lengthy audit, and my relationship was crumbling. My high school sweetheart came to terms with something he'd been quietly wrestling with, and it meant our story was ending. Supporting him through that while trying to understand myself was its own kind of heartbreak.

Then came what textbooks might politely call a "nervous breakdown." In reality, it looked like crying on the hardwood floor at 2 a.m., bargaining with a maybe-God for one night of peace. My body shook, my brain sprinted, and I remember wondering if minds could actually short-circuit, because I'm almost certain mine was doing so. What I didn't know then was that my amygdala (the brain's alarm system) was doing its job a little too well. When the body senses threat, real or emotional, it floods itself with cortisol and adrenaline. Logic exits the chat. Your pulse races, your stomach knots, and your thoughts turn into static. It's simply chemistry. And I was drowning in it and suddenly couldn't think straight long enough to calm down. I wasn't crazy. I was chemically cornered and neurologically trapped.

And when your brain feels trapped, it starts looking for exits, any exits. That's how I stumbled into distraction disguised as freedom. I went full-throttle party mode. Raves, festivals, after-parties that turned into before-work parties. I was basically powered by Red Bull, glitter, and emotional avoidance. I'd dance until sunrise, stumble home, shower, and clock in like nothing happened. Functional? Technically. Fulfilled? Absolutely not. That's the dangerous part about functioning: It tricks everyone, especially you, into thinking you're okay.

I kept surrounding myself with people who didn't quite sit right in my soul but they were loud enough to drown out the silence. And the silence was what terrified me. Because when the music stopped, I had to be alone with my own thoughts. And that was scarier than any hangover.

So I filled the quiet with noise, hours of news, endless reels, partying, and every *Real Housewives* franchise known to humankind. I'd scroll through Instagram and Hulu thinking, *What's wrong with me? Why does everyone else seem so happy, so energetic, while I just feel . . . flat?*

It was a slow-motion meltdown because silence had become something I feared. When, really, it was the only place I could've met myself.

Fear robs us of happiness like that. It convinces us that stillness is dangerous, that if we stop moving, all the noise inside will swallow us whole. But the truth? Stillness is where the real healing hides.

One of my favorite psychologist friends told me that mid-breakdown.

I hung up on her, obviously. Who wants philosophy when they're falling apart?

But again, hindsight is twenty-twenty.

There's only so long your nervous system can sprint before it face-plants. Eventually, I hit a wall. Not a dramatic crash, but that quiet, creeping kind of *not okay.*

I was what I now call a "slippery patient."

Functional, absent. Not in crisis, but far from fine.

Tired of being tired. Burned out on surviving.

Trying to rewire the neural chaos that had become my default setting. And for a while, it helped. I found tools. Language. Glimmers of peace. But healing isn't linear. And just when you think you've got it handled, the universe throws you a final boss.

For me, that boss wore a familiar name: SSRIs. The same antidepressant class of drugs I was prescribed at sixteen. The one I turned to again in my thirties when things got dark. Except this time, it didn't help. It nearly wrecked me.

My inner voice didn't feel like mine anymore.

Not in a poetic, soft-focus kind of way.

In a "Do I need to check myself into a facility?" kind of way.

In a "This twelfth-story balcony is starting to look like an exit" kind of way.

That was my line in the sand, the moment I realized survival had to become a skill, not an accident, and biology doesn't care about good intentions.

The reckoning.

The no-more-BS, get-serious-about-myself moment.

Because no one was coming to save me, and this wasn't something I could fix with a prescription and a planner.

So I got to work.

On me.

Not because I loved myself yet.

Not because I felt ready.

But because I finally understood the cost of not trying.

That's why this book exists, because the systems built to help us heal were never designed for women like us in the first place and feel more like a Band-Aid on a broken leg than real, sustainable tools. The post-pandemic world left us more disconnected, more depleted, and more gaslit than ever. Women are being diagnosed with ADHD, anxiety, premenstrual dysphoric disorder (PMDD), OCD (me), and other mental health complications in record numbers, and we're told to relax, journal, and maybe download another meditation app, while our hormones scream for nutrients and our nervous systems fray like cheap cable cords.

I'm not a therapist. I'm not here to diagnose or prescribe. I'm just a scientist with a browser history full of panic-induced Google searches, who decided to get uncomfortably curious about what actually helps. I'm also a dog mom with a borderline obsessive love for my fur babies, a wife to a man who somehow cracked the code to my mental health (he's a saint, truly), and a lifelong card-carrying member of the Anxiety Club. Here at your service.

One final word before we get started, on what you'll find in the pages that follow. This book is built on what I call the Load Capacity Framework. Think of your nervous system like your phone battery. When it's at 100 percent, you can handle anything: stressful meetings, emotional challenges, daily chaos. But when your battery is at 15 percent? Everything becomes overwhelming. The difference is your load capacity. Your nervous system has a certain amount of capacity to handle stress, process emotions, and make decisions. When that capacity is depleted, everything feels harder because you're biologically overloaded.

Here's what most people miss: Load capacity is biological. If your iron is low, your brain isn't getting enough oxygen. That's load. If your thyroid is sluggish, your neurons fire slower. That's load. If you're deficient in magnesium, your nervous system can't downregulate. That's load. Throughout this book, you'll learn to recognize your Clinical Cues (the signals your body sends when load capacity is compromised) and match them to what's actually happening in your biology. You can't meditate your way out of iron deficiency, and you can't journal your way out of hypothyroidism. Let's restore your capacity at the biological level and address symptoms at their source.

# WHAT YOU'LL GET

## 🧠 Chapter-End Recaps to Keep It Simple

After each chapter, you'll find a mini-chapter called "TL;DR, Do This Now, and Clinical Cues." It will give you:

- The brain-friendly CliffsNotes version
- Tiny, doable steps to put the information into action (a.k.a. the bare minimum)
- The clinical tests to request and how to ask your doctor for them

That's right. No thirty-day challenges or toxic productivity hacks. Just the smallest possible thing you can do today to move the needle.

## Summaries

We'll also summarize each of the book's five parts when we get to the end. Because this book is here to help you, not give you more homework.

## The Game Plan: What's in Each Part

### Part 1: You Are What You Eat

Nutrients matter. A lot. Especially the ones your doctor forgot to mention while telling you you're "fine." We'll cover the biological foundations of mental wellness, from omega-3s and B12 to the gut–brain axis and why your takeout habit isn't helping.

## Part 2: Your Hormones, Your Cycle

We'll cover your menstrual cycle as a monthly neurochemical event, the perimenopause transition nobody warned you about, menopause and what it actually does to your brain, and the thyroid gland that controls whether any of it runs at full speed. If you've ever been told your labs are "normal" while you felt anything but, this part is your proof that you were right.

## Part 3: Move Your Mind—The Science and Soul of Sweat

Movement isn't punishment; it's your brain's favorite antidepressant. Learn how exercise (even the lazy kind) can rewire your neurochemistry, lift your mood, and get you unstuck.

## Part 4: Because Even Your Brain Needs a Group Chat

Loneliness is a bigger threat than carbs. We'll explore why community isn't just nice; it's necessary. You don't need thirty-seven best friends. You need connection that feeds you.

## Part 5: Mind Over Matter (and Mood): The Case for Mindfulness in a Chaotic World

Mindfulness without the eye roll. From Buddhism to Stoicism to trauma-informed presence, we'll explore the neuroscience of awareness and how to actually calm the chaos.

## Part 6: Do Something Useless: The Life-Saving Magic of Hobbies

No, you don't need to monetize your joy. You need to do something useless for your brain, your identity, and your sanity. We'll break down the psychology of play, creativity, and rest that isn't performative.

If you've ever looked at your life and whispered, "How do I fix this, even just a little?" you're exactly the kind of person this book was written for.

You don't need another productivity system. You need nourishment. Restoration. A plan that works with your biology, not against it.

This isn't a self-help book; it's the manual you were supposed to get at birth. Let's begin.

# PART 1

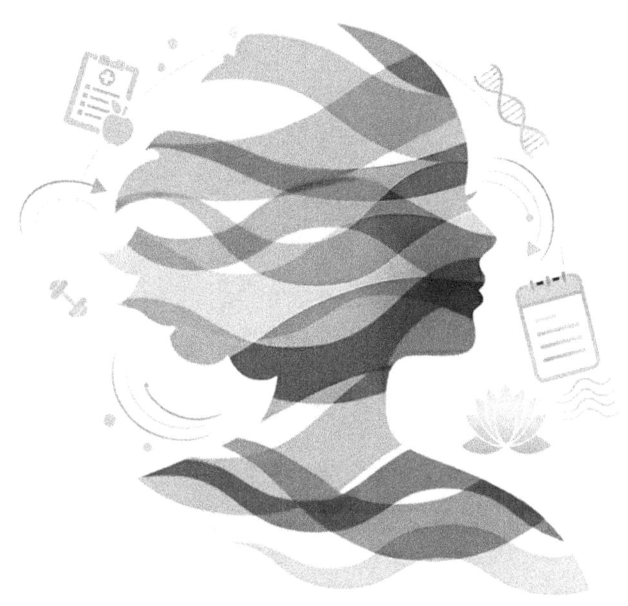

# YOU ARE WHAT YOU EAT

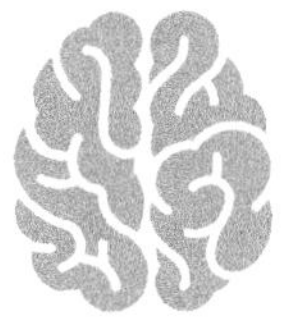



# CHAPTER 2

# THE FATTY ACID TRIP: OMEGA-3S AND THE BRAINY SIDE OF FATS

## Omega-3s: Your Brain's Favorite Fuel

Your brain runs the whole show, burning more energy than any other organ and demanding premium fuel to function. Skimp on quality, and you get emotional instability, constant overthinking, and performance issues. Enter omega-3 fatty acids, the architects and structural engineers your brain needs to stay stable. These fats are elite. Imagine them in velvet tracksuits, sipping green juice and expecting optimal neuron performance at all times. They build the brain, tame inflammation, and help brain cells communicate, keeping the group chat alive instead of ghosting like my therapist once did. Without enough omega-3s, your brain is basically trying to run a marathon in flip-flops.

And that's a hard no.

There are three main types of omega-3s, and each one plays a distinct role in the brain:

Alpha-linolenic acid (ALA) is the plant-based omega-3 you'll find in flaxseeds, chia seeds, walnuts, and hemp seeds. It's the gateway omega-3, the one you can easily get through food. But here's the catch: It doesn't convert into the other omega-3s (EPA and DHA) very efficiently. Your body only turns about 5–10 percent of ALA into EPA, and less than 1 percent into DHA. It's like going to Olive Garden, ordering lasagna, and they only bring you the breadsticks. Cute, but not even close to what you came for. While ALA is essential (you can't make it on your own), serious brain support requires direct EPA and DHA. Direct sources of EPA and DHA, usually from fatty fish or algae-based supplements, are the real MVPs. Your body tries to turn ALA into EPA and DHA, but the process is hilariously inefficient. A few things make conversion better: enough zinc, B6, and magnesium, plus low inflammation. A few things tank conversion: chronic stress, drinking too much, and inflammation. Women generally convert ALA better than men, thanks to estrogen, but even then, it's nowhere near the amount your brain actually wants. Which is why relying on ALA alone is the nutritional equivalent of expecting a Sunday girls' brunch to stay calm during Mercury retrograde. It's just not going to happen. DHA and EPA do the heavy lifting when it comes to supporting your neurons, keeping your brain cells fluid and talkative, and calming inflammation.

Eicosapentaenoic acid (EPA) comes from fatty fish-like salmon, sardines, mackerel, anchovies, and herring. It's the facilities manager clearing out inflammatory disruptions before they shut down operations, producing signaling molecules called eicosanoids that regulate immune responses and calm inflammatory chaos. In the brain, that anti-inflammatory power translates to lower risk of mood disorders and slower cognitive decline.

Unlike some fats that mostly become part of cell membranes and just hang out as structural wallpaper, EPA doesn't stay on the sidelines. It's active. It gets used, quickly, in the chemical pathways that dial inflammation up or down. That's what I mean by it not just sitting around as "structural wallpaper."

Clinical studies [shoutout to Sublette et al. (2011) in *The Journal of Clinical Psychiatry*] show that higher EPA intake correlates with improved mood and fewer symptoms of major depressive disorder. For people with elevated inflammation markers like CRP (C-Reactive Protein) or IL-6 (Interleukin-6), EPA can be especially powerful. Some researchers even recommend pairing EPA with antidepressants for better results.

If EPA is your inflammation warrior, DHA is the architect. One keeps the peace; the other builds the city. Docosahexaenoic acid (DHA) is the structural royalty of brain fats. Also found in fatty fish and high-quality supplements, DHA makes up about 25 percent of the fat in your brain's gray matter and 60 percent of the polyunsaturated fatty acids in your neurons. It's all about keeping your brain nimble, sharp, and communicative. Thanks to its six double bonds (hello, flexible molecule), DHA helps your neurons stay fluid, which boosts everything from memory to mood regulation. DHA also helps regulate the emotional circuitry between the amygdala (your alarm system) and the prefrontal cortex (your reasoning). When DHA is low, that communication gets glitchy, so stress feels louder, irritation sits closer to the surface, and your emotional reactions fire faster than you want. Women also tend to need more DHA during major hormonal phases. Estrogen boosts DHA retention, but hormonal birth control, perimenopause, pregnancy, and chronic stress all drain it. That's one reason many women feel mentally sharper and more emotionally steady when their omega-3 intake improves. Furthermore, deficiencies in DHA are associated with cognitive decline, including conditions like Alzheimer's. A clinical study by Yurko-Mauro et al. (2010) in *Alzheimer's & Dementia®* showed that DHA supplementation can improve cognitive function in older adults. Bottom line: A well-fed brain is a smart brain.

## Why It Matters for Your Mental Health

Omega-3s don't just influence your brain; they talk directly to your hormones. They help stabilize cortisol rhythms, reduce prostaglandins that cause painful periods, and improve communication between hormone receptors. Many women notice smoother PMS symptoms, more stable mood during cycle shifts, and fewer emotional land mines when omega-3 intake is consistent. This happens because cell membranes finally have the raw material they need. Omega-3s build your brain, literally. They make up a significant portion of neural tissue. They also tone down neuroinflammation, which is the sneaky villain who's always somewhere behind the scenes of anxiety, depression, and general fogginess. Plus, they support the production of neurotransmitters like serotonin and dopamine. If those names sound familiar, it's because they're your brain's mood managers.

Some studies even suggest that EPA-heavy supplements work just as well as antidepressants for mild to moderate depression, without the typical side effects. [Freeman et al. (2006) *The American Journal of Psychiatry*] Translation? You could be a few fish dinners away from feeling more balanced.

The easiest way to show your brain some love? Eat fatty fish two to three times per week. Salmon, sardines, anchovies, and mackerel are loaded with both EPA and DHA. Plant based? No problem. Chia seeds, flaxseeds, hemp seeds, and walnuts can boost your ALA intake. But remember, ALA doesn't convert very well, so a high-quality algae-based supplement is a smart move if fish is off the table.

When choosing a supplement, read beyond the flashy front label. Look at the actual amounts of EPA and DHA per serving; that's what your brain cares about. Aim for 500 to 1,000 mg of combined EPA and DHA daily for general brain support.

---

## EXPERT SIDEBAR:
### "Not All Omega-3 Supplements Are Created Equal"

Let's be real. Not all omega-3s are worth your time (or your money). Look for ones labeled as triglyceride or re-esterified triglyceride form, these are easier to absorb than the cheaper ethyl ester versions. Make sure the brand does third-party testing for purity, potency, and no heavy metals. If you're vegan, go for algae oil with both EPA and DHA in meaningful amounts. And don't forget: Consistency is key. Omega-3s need time to build up in your system to work their full magic. One pill won't do it. This is a long game.

---

## Let's Hit Pause

That was a fatty-acid crash course, and now your brain deserves a quick summary. Whether you're reading this on the go or just need the straight-to-the-point version, the next section is your shortcut to the essentials and your action plan.

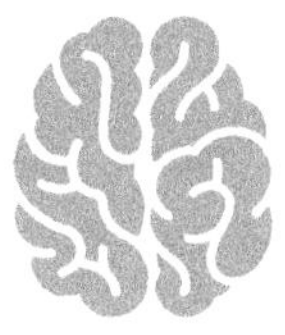



# TL;DR, DO THIS NOW, AND CLINICAL CUES

## ☑ TL;DR

Omega-3s are the fuel your brain is begging for. ALA is the plant-based rookie, EPA is the inflammation fixer, and DHA is the structural queen that keeps your neurons agile and your mind sharp. Without enough of these fats, your brain is working overtime on low power mode. Mood issues, mental fog, and lack of focus are all common signs your system needs a fatty-acid upgrade.

## ☑ Do This Now

Pick one step and do it today. Add a fatty fish (salmon, sardines, mackerel) to your next meal plan or grab a high-quality algae-based supplement with 500 to 1,000 mg of combined EPA and DHA. Check the label for real amounts. If you're more of a smoothie or salad person, toss in flaxseeds, walnuts, or chia for bonus ALA. Make it a habit, not a heroic one-time effort. This is about building brain resilience bite by bite.

## ☑ Clinical Cues

This short guide helps you understand how to read lab ranges the way a clinician or scientist does. "Normal" reflects the broad lab reference interval, while "Optimal" shows the range where most women feel and function their best. Use these "Clinical Cues" to understand your own labs and when a value that's "technically fine" might still be dragging down your mood, sleep, or energy.

### ▪ Omega-3 Index (EPA and DHA Percent of total fatty acids)

- Normal: ≥4 percent
- Optimal: 8–12 percent

**What this actually means:** When you get your Omega-3 Index tested, the lab measures the percentage of EPA and DHA in your red blood cell membranes.

That number usually lands somewhere between 2 and 12 percent. The higher the percentage, the more omega-3s your cells have available for anti-inflammatory signaling and brain health.

A normal result is anything at or above 4 percent. It's not dangerous, but it's not where mood or cognition tend to thrive.

An optimal range is 8 to 12 percent, which is where research shows the most consistent benefits for lowering neuroinflammation, stabilizing mood, and supporting focus and emotional resilience.

**Why it matters:** Low omega-3 status is linked to higher baseline inflammation. Women with low levels are more likely to experience postpartum depression, perimenopausal mood shifts, and stress-resistant anxiety. EPA helps lower neuroinflammation and supports serotonin signaling; DHA strengthens neuronal membranes and improves communication between brain regions. If you're dealing with brain fog, dry skin, or mood changes (especially in your luteal phase), this lab is a quiet instigator.

If you want more targeted support, think about dosing like this:

- **Mood support:** 1,000 to 2,000 mg daily, with EPA dominant
- **PMS/PMDD:** EPA-heavy blends work best for inflammation-driven mood swings.
- **Cognitive support:** DHA-forward formulas
- **Inflammation:** EPA > DHA

These aren't hard rules, but they help your brain get the right tool for the job.

### ▨ **Triglycerides**

- Normal: <150 mg/dL
- Optimal: <100 mg/dL

**Why it matters:** High triglycerides = poor omega-3 intake + possible insulin resistance. In women, this often shows up as fatigue, difficulty losing weight after age thirty-five, or more severe PMS. Low triglycerides plus a high Omega-3 Index? That's the brain-protective combo.

## ☑ Moving On

Now that your brain has its essential fats in place and is starting to think straight again, it's time to support the crew behind the scenes. Enter the B vitamins, your internal energy engineers, neurotransmitter technicians, and hormone harmonizers. If omega-3s get your neurons chatting, the Bs make sure they show up on time, say the right thing, and don't light anything on fire. In Chapter 3, we're diving into the nutrient trio that can transform fatigue, mood swings, and monthly meltdowns into something a lot more manageable.

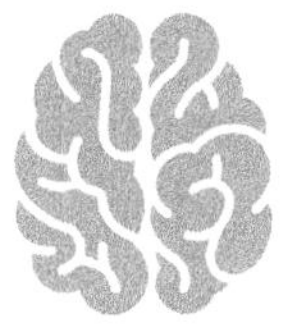



# HARDER, BETTER, FASTER, STRONGER: THE B TEAM (B6, FOLATE, B12, MTHFR, PMS SUPPORT)

If omega-3s are the architects of your brain, B vitamins are the construction crew, electricians, and maintenance team. This water-soluble power crew keeps your brain humming on every level.

They help build neurotransmitters, repair DNA, and convert food into cellular energy. And here's the real headline and why it's important here: Most people have no idea that they are low on these mood-boosting micronutrients.

Let's break down the big hitters.

## Vitamin B6 (Pyridoxine): The Neurotransmitter Whisperer

Vitamin B6 is essential for synthesizing serotonin, dopamine, and GABA, the trio of chemical messengers that regulate mood, motivation, and sleep. Low levels of B6 are linked to irritability, depression, anxiety, and even cognitive dysfunction.

Pro tip: B6 is heat sensitive. Light steaming is fine, but boiling or overcooking can wipe out its benefits.

- Best sources: bananas, chickpeas, salmon, turkey, sweet potatoes, and fortified cereals

## Vitamin B9 (Folate): The Methylation Powerhouse

Folate (in its natural form) and folic acid (synthetic form) play major roles in one-carbon metabolism. Folate is the city planner of your brain. It signs off on new buildings, repairs damaged roads, and keeps traffic flowing so your cells can detox, repair, and make neurotransmitters. It also keeps homocysteine, an inflammatory marker linked to depression and Alzheimer's, in check. Low folate equals a higher risk of depression and lowered responsivity to antidepressants.

- Best sources: leafy greens like spinach, romaine, and kale, plus lentils, asparagus, and avocados

## Vitamin B12 (Cobalamin): The Brain-Fog Buster

Vitamin B12 supports nerve health, red blood cell production, and DNA synthesis. Deficiency can lead to fatigue, memory lapses, mood swings, and even tingling in the extremities. Vegans and vegetarians are especially at risk since B12 is mostly found in animal products.

- Best sources: beef liver, sardines, eggs, nutritional yeast, dairy, and fortified plant milks

---

### EXPERT SIDEBAR:
### Why You Might Still Be Deficient

"Stress, alcohol, birth control pills, aging, and gut issues (like IBS or low stomach acid) can all deplete B vitamins or interfere with absorption, even if your diet seems pretty good. If you're chronically tired, foggy, or moody, a B complex might be your new best friend."
—A Clinical Nutritionist Somewhere Between Science Nerd and Realist

---

## A Quick Note on Supplementation

If you're considering supplements, go for a methylated B complex. Not all supplements are created equal, and your body doesn't just magically activate nutrients on its own, especially if you're dealing with genetic roadblocks, stress, or gut imbalances. Methylated forms of B12 (methylcobalamin) and folate (methylfolate) are already in the active form your body uses, which makes them far more effective. If your multivitamin just says "folic acid" or "cyanocobalamin," you might be taking in nutrients that your body can't fully use, which is kind of like pouring premium fuel into a car that doesn't have a working engine.

Also, don't forget that timing and pairing matter. Take your B complex with food to reduce the chance of nausea or lightheadedness, especially if you're sensitive to energy shifts. Morning is usually best; some people feel a gentle boost from Bs and don't want to be wired at bedtime. And be consistent. These vitamins are water soluble, meaning your body doesn't store them long term. A missed day here and there won't ruin your progress, but regular intake builds the foundation your nervous system needs.

If you've been burning the candle at both ends, skipping meals, or feeling like your emotions are on a roller coaster, your body is practically begging for some nutritional backup. A quality B complex can be that quiet, behind-the-scenes helper that keeps everything in check.

It's especially important to choose a methylated B complex if you have genetic variations like MTHFR. What's MTHFR?

Glad you asked.

## MTHFR: The Genetic Plot Twist

MTHFR (methylenetetrahydrofolate reductase, say that three times fast) is a gene involved in processing folate and B12. Roughly

40 percent of people have a variant that slows this process down. This means your body may not activate these nutrients effectively, even if you're getting them through food.

Signs of sluggish methylation: anxiety, irritability, hormone imbalance, fatigue, and weirdly brutal hangovers. Look for supplements with active forms like methylcobalamin (B12) and methylfolate (B9) and always pair them with food to avoid nausea.

## What the Science Says

Vitamin B12 is critical for red blood cell production, neurological function, and energy metabolism, all of which can get thrown off by your menstrual cycle. Low B12, especially when combined with low folate or B6, has been linked to more intense PMS symptoms and impaired estrogen detox in the liver. Translation? Hormonal chaos.

One 2023 study found that women who took B-complex vitamins (including B12) had significant improvements in mood stability, fatigue, and anxiety during their cycle compared to a placebo group [Borges-Vieira & Cardoso, Nutritional Neuroscience, 2023].

## B12 Saved Me from the Period Pit of Despair

For months, like clockwork, my luteal phase would roll in and absolutely flatten me. I'm talking bone-deep exhaustion, thick brain fog, and snapping at someone over absolutely nothing. It didn't feel like regular PMS; it felt like a full system power-down.

After some trial and error (and a tip from a nerdy friend), I got my B12 levels checked. Turns out, I was technically "within range" but nowhere near optimal. I started supplementing with methylcobalamin, and by the second cycle, it felt like someone had flipped the lights back on. My mood steadied. I had energy. I didn't need a nap, three motivational podcasts, and a pep talk from my dog just to make it through the day.

I still get cramps. I still want to throat-punch capitalism once a month. But I no longer feel like I'm drowning. And that's a massive win.

## Cycle-Linked Brain States: Why Your Mood and Cognition Shift Week to Week

Your brain chemistry doesn't stay constant across the month. Estrogen, progesterone, inflammation patterns, insulin sensitivity, neurotransmitter balance, and micronutrient utilization all change as your cycle moves through its phases.

These shifts alter how your brain processes stress, regulates emotion, and maintains cognitive clarity. Call it what it is: physiology.

What that means on the ground level:

**Follicular Phase (post-period to ovulation):**
Estrogen rises, which increases serotonin signaling, sharpens synaptic efficiency, boosts verbal fluency, and improves emotional tolerance. Most women feel more stable, resilient, and cognitively sharp here.

**Luteal Phase (after ovulation):**

Progesterone increases GABA activity for calm and sleep support, but insulin sensitivity dips, inflammation markers can rise, and serotonin availability drops in susceptible women. If micronutrient stores are low, especially iron, magnesium, zinc, B6, or omega-3s, this phase amplifies anxiety, irritability, cravings, brain fog, and emotional sensitivity.

**Late Luteal Phase (PMS window):**

This is where ferritin deficits, low DHA, poor sleep, and unstable glucose pull the floor out from under your mood. The brain runs "hotter": Cortisol spikes, rumination rises, inflammatory tone worsens, and neurotransmitter production becomes less efficient. That emotional intensity? Lower metabolic cushioning at work.

Micronutrients tie directly into this pattern:

- B vitamins drive neurotransmitter synthesis.
- Omega-3s reduce inflammatory load and stabilize serotonin signaling.
- Magnesium and zinc support GABA function.
- Ferritin determines oxygen supply and dopamine activity.

When these reserves are full, the hormonal shifts feel like subtle background noise.

When they're depleted, the exact same shifts hit harder and feel like emotional upheaval.

Your experience isn't random.

Your brain is responding to chemistry it didn't choose and inputs it hasn't always had.

This is why nutrition, sleep depth, iron stores, Omega-3 Index, anti-inflammatory patterns, and stable blood sugar matter. They make the difference between a turbulent luteal week and one that feels grounded, tolerable, and emotionally coherent.

Your brain isn't changing every month.

Its operating environment is.

Support the environment, and the emotional waves flatten.

## Bottom Line

B vitamins are essential, not optional. If your mood is shaky, your energy's tanked, or PMS is out here acting like a wrecking ball, your nervous system might be starved for support. Give it the B-team backup it deserves.

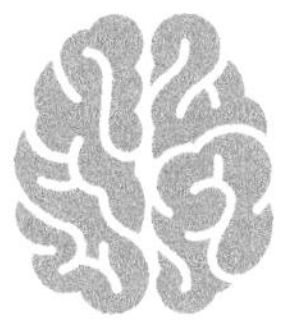



# TL;DR, DO THIS NOW, AND CLINICAL CUES

## ☑ TL;DR

B vitamins are like a support staff for your entire mental and hormonal system. B6 keeps neurotransmitters flowing, folate keeps things clean and detoxified, and B12 sharpens memory and energy while saving your sanity during PMS. Modern life, stress, and genetics can all drain these nutrients, leaving you foggy, anxious, and fried.

## ☑ Do This Now

Start with a methylated B-complex supplement that includes B6, methylfolate, and methylcobalamin. Check your labels and look for food-based or activated forms. If you're plant based, make sure B12 is covered. Add more leafy greens, lentils, eggs, and fortified foods to your plate this week. And if your cycle knocks you flat every month, get your B levels tested. Your future self will high-five you.

## ☑ Clinical Cues

### ▨ Vitamin B12 (serum)

- Normal: 200–900 pg/mL
  This is the reference range labs use. Anything above 200 technically counts as "normal," but it doesn't mean your brain is actually happy here.

- Optimal: 500–800 pg/mL
  This is the range where most people *feel* their best. Mood, energy, hair, focus, and nerve function all tend to stabilize when B12 is comfortably in the middle rather than scraping the bottom.

**Why it matters:** B12 deficiency often hides under the label "low normal," which is medical shorthand for "You're technically fine, but you feel like garbage." Women in their twenties to sixties with low B12 report fatigue, thinning hair, brain fog, anxiety, and more intense PMS. Diets low in animal products, metformin, gut issues, and birth control can all reduce B12 absorption.

### ▪ Vitamin B6

- Normal: 5-50 mcg/L (varies by lab)
- Optimal: 20-50 mcg/L

**Why it matters:** Low B6 = impaired serotonin and GABA synthesis, worse PMS, increased anxiety. Women on oral contraceptives are at higher risk for depletion.

### ▪ Estradiol (E2)

Reference varies by cycle phase.

- Follicular: 30-120 pg/mL
- Mid-cycle: 100-400 pg/mL
- Luteal: 50-250 pg/mL

### ▪ Progesterone (mid-luteal):

- Normal: 2-25 ng/mL (luteal)
- Optimal: 10-25 ng/mL mid-luteal

**When to test:** Mid-luteal for progesterone; day three of cycle for FSH/E2.

**Why it matters:** Low progesterone = luteal phase anxiety + insomnia. High estrogen relative to progesterone = PMS rage, heavy periods, migraines.

### Testosterone (total, female):

- Normal: 15-70 ng/dL
- Optimal: 30-60 ng/dL

### Free Testosterone (female):

- Normal: 0.1-6.4 pg/mL

**Why it matters:** Low testosterone = fatigue, low libido, loss of drive. High testosterone = PCOS signs like acne and irregular cycles.

### Sex Hormone Binding Globulin:

- Normal: 18-144 nmol/L
- Optimal: 60-80 nmol/L

**Why it matters:** Tied to metabolic health and estrogen balance. Low SHBG = PCOS, high androgens, insulin resistance. High SHBG = low free testosterone, fatigue, low libido.

### Pregnenolone (serum)

**Why it matters:** "Mother hormone." Low levels = brain fog, poor memory, perimenopausal mood swings. Stress depletes it.

### ▨ Estrone (E1)

**Why it matters:** Often overlooked estrogen fraction. In perimenopause and postmenopause, estrone dominance relative to estradiol can drive mood instability, hot flashes, and metabolic shifts.

### ▨ Methylmalonic Acid (MMA)

- Normal: <0.4 μmol/L

**Why it matters:** Elevated MMA = your cells are starving for B12, even if your serum looks fine. This is why some women with "normal" labs still feel like zombies.

### ▨ Homocysteine

- Normal: 5–15 μmol/L
- Optimal: 6–9 μmol/L

**Why it matters:** Elevated homocysteine is a red flag for sluggish methylation, the process that drives neurotransmitter production, detoxing estrogen, and even fertility. Women with high homocysteine often struggle with anxiety, recurrent miscarriages, and perimenopausal mood instability.

### ▪ RBC Folate

- Normal: >200 ng/mL
- Optimal: >400 ng/mL

**Why it matters:** Folate keeps estrogen metabolism on track and reduces PMS severity. Low folate = worse mood swings around ovulation and luteal phase.

## ☑ Moving On

Now that your brain's running more smoothly thanks to the B-vitamin dream team, it's time to zoom out and look at the bigger picture because mood and focus aren't just about neurotransmitters. They're also deeply tied to your hormones, minerals, and your body's ability to handle stress without imploding. In Chapter 4, we're bringing in the sunshine (literally) and rounding up the mineral squad: vitamin D, zinc, magnesium, iron, and the antioxidant defenders who protect your brain from biochemical drama. If your nervous system still feels like it's on a reality show called *Barely Coping,* this next part is for you.

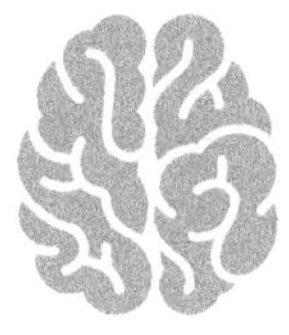



# VITAMIN D, THE MINERAL SQUAD, AND OXIDATIVE STRESS (D3, ZINC, MAGNESIUM, IRON, ANTIOXIDANT DEFENSE)

## Vitamin D: The Sunshine Boss of Mood and Immunity

If B vitamins are the construction crew, vitamin D is the zoning commissioner, regulating what gets built, when, and how the immune system patrols the neighborhood. Despite its name, vitamin D is actually a hormone that regulates mood stability, cognitive function, and inflammation.

So what does it actually do?

*Mood stabilizer:* Low vitamin D levels have been linked to depression, seasonal mood swings, and chronic blah syndrome. It helps regulate serotonin, the same mood chemical targeted by many antidepressants. The connection holds year-round, not just during winter. Studies consistently show that low vitamin D is associated with an increased risk of depression, whether it's seasonal or not. A 2013 meta-analysis published in *The British Journal of Psychiatry* found that individuals with low vitamin D levels were more than twice as likely to experience depression. The connection is strong, widespread, and too important to ignore.

*Brain builder:* Vitamin D supports neuroplasticity, which is your brain's ability to adapt, rewire, and bounce back from mental overload. It also helps reduce inflammation, a major contributor to emotional and cognitive wear and tear.

*Immune regulator:* It keeps your immune system alert without making it paranoid. Think of it as the calm, experienced bouncer at the immune system's door: firm but fair.

Where can you get it?

- Sunlight: About fifteen to twenty minutes of direct sun exposure can help your body make its own D, but this varies depending on your location, skin tone, season, and sunscreen because yes, the SPF that protects your skin also blocks the UV you need for vitamin D.
- Food sources: fatty fish (salmon, sardines), egg yolks, fortified plant milks and cereals

- Supplements: Often necessary, especially if you're not getting consistent sun exposure. Look for D3 (cholecalciferol), which is more bioavailable than D2.

Translation: If you've been stuck in a rut, can't remember the last time you felt energized, or the winter blues hit like a freight train every year, get your D levels checked. You might be biologically craving sunlight, not just a vacation.

So what's optimal? While most labs consider anything over 30 ng/mL to be "normal," that's the bare minimum to avoid deficiency-related disease. For optimal brain and immune function, many functional medicine practitioners recommend keeping your serum 25(OH)D levels between 50 and 70 ng/mL. If you've struggled with chronic fatigue, immune issues, or depression, aiming for the higher end of that range can make a noticeable difference.

## Zinc, Magnesium, and Iron

Your brain is basically a high-maintenance chemical lab, constantly producing neurotransmitters, the mood messengers that keep you focused, calm, and emotionally steady. But these messengers don't make themselves. They need building blocks, and key minerals like zinc, magnesium, and iron play leading roles.

### Zinc: The Quiet Mood Stabilizer

Zinc is involved in producing and regulating GABA (your chill-out neurotransmitter) and glutamate (your learning and memory booster). It's the brain's quality control agent, keeping excitability in check and preventing burnout on the molecular level. Low zinc is consistently linked with mood disorders and even treatment-resistant depression. Supplementing with zinc has been shown to enhance the effectiveness of antidepressants.

- Food sources: oysters, pumpkin seeds, cashews, beef

**Magnesium: The Nervous System's Wingwoman**
Magnesium is the cofactor for converting tryptophan (a precursor to serotonin) into its usable form. Without it, your serotonin production slows down, leaving your mood hanging.

It also binds to GABA receptors, which is why it's often recommended for anxiety and better sleep. Stress burns through magnesium fast, so if you're chronically overwhelmed, chances are your levels are depleted.

- Food sources: leafy greens, almonds, black beans, avocado, and dark chocolate (yes, permission granted)

**Iron: The Energy and Focus MVP**
Iron is essential for synthesizing dopamine (motivation, reward, pleasure) and serotonin (mood and emotional regulation). It also helps oxygenate the brain—kind of important for, well, thinking. Low iron is linked to brain fog, fatigue, low motivation, and even increased anxiety. It's particularly crucial for menstruating individuals.

- Food sources: red meat, lentils, tofu, spinach. Pair plant-based iron with vitamin C (like citrus or bell peppers) to boost absorption.

These three minerals also work together: Zinc and magnesium balance neurotransmitter activity, and magnesium and iron power the energy production required to make those neurotransmitters in the first place. But don't overdo it; too much zinc can block iron absorption, so balance is key.

## The Chaos Magnet of Your Brain: Oxidative Stress and Mental Health

Let's talk about oxidative stress, the biochemical chaos magnet of your nervous system. It shows up when unstable molecules called free radicals start trashing your brain cells. Normally, antioxidants play cleanup crew and restore order. But when you're running low on antioxidants (or high on stress and processed food), those free radicals party like they've got nothing to lose. Cue inflammation, scrambled neurotransmitters, and a welcome mat for anxiety, depression, and brain fog.

Modern life amplifies this beyond individual habits. Undersleeping, stress-looping, eating nutrient-depleted junk, doomscrolling instead of de-stressing? All of it fuels oxidative stress. And when antioxidants like vitamins C and E don't show up to neutralize the free radicals damaging your cells, the mental mess accumulates fast.

## Clinical Logic for Symptoms: How to Read What Your Brain Is Asking For

Symptoms are information your body is giving you. When something feels off like mood, energy, cravings, anxiety, fog, irritability, it usually means one of the core biological drivers is under-resourced. When you understand those drivers, you can respond like a clinician rather than with self-blame.

Here's the simplest diagnostic logic to start with:

**If you feel wired-tired, overwhelmed, or anxious:**
- Check sleep depth and magnesium status.

Low magnesium, fragmented sleep, and high cortisol all make your brain run "hot," pushing your nervous system toward rumination, vigilance, rapid thoughts, and irritability. Prioritize evening sleep hygiene, magnesium glycinate, and a protein-rich breakfast to stabilize cortisol.

**If you feel brain-foggy, apathetic, low-motivation, or fatigued:**
- Look at ferritin, Omega-3 Index, and vitamin D.

Low ferritin robs neurons of oxygen and tanks dopamine signaling. Low omega-3 raises inflammatory tone and dulls serotonin sensitivity. Low vitamin D impacts mood circuitry and neuroplasticity. Supporting these often clears the fog more than any mindset technique.

**If cravings, mood drops, or irritability spike in the luteal phase:**
- Think inflammation and micronutrient demand.

Progesterone changes insulin sensitivity, shifts neurotransmitter balance, and raises inflammatory load. Iron deficits, omega-3 insufficiency, and low magnesium make that shift hit harder. Support ferritin, stabilize glucose, and increase DHA.

**If mood swings hit after a bad week of sleep, stress, or processed food:**
- It's likely inflammatory overshoot.

CRP, cytokine release, and glucose swings directly alter serotonin, dopamine, and GABA tone. Go back to fiber, whole nutrients, early circadian alignment, and light movement.

**If you feel depressed, shut down, irritated at everyone, or emotionally fragile:**
- Scan for under-recovery.

Sleep depth, ferritin stores, glucose stability, and omega-3 availability determine your load capacity. When those are thin, emotional weight feels heavier than it "should." Refuel, restore sleep, and regulate blood sugar before you go into existential crisis.

**If intrusive thoughts spike at night:**
- Check evening glucose behavior and magnesium.

Nighttime neuroinflammation and cortisol residuals worsen cognitive rumination. Magnesium, stable blood sugar, and earlier meals often help more than willpower.

None of these patterns are moral evaluations.

They're resource equations.

You were never meant to make sense of your mental world without understanding your biological one.

Use these patterns as reflection prompts, not diagnoses. They offer direction rather than labels. And as you learn your own rhythms, this becomes second nature and curiosity replaces panic; troubleshooting replaces self-judgment.

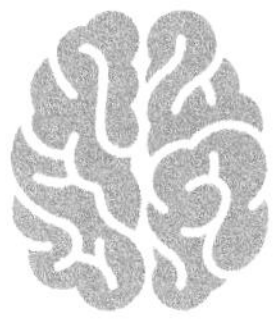



# TL;DR, DO THIS NOW, AND CLINICAL CUES

## ☑ TL;DR

Vitamin D is your neuro-immune heavy hitter, zinc keeps your mood in check, magnesium supports calm and sleep, and iron fuels motivation and brainpower. They are all team players in the brain's neurotransmitter orchestra. Meanwhile, oxidative stress is the chaos agent; you need antioxidants and lifestyle support to keep it in line.

## ☑ Do This Now

Book a quick blood test to check your vitamin D and iron levels (especially if you feel constantly tired or blue). Add fatty fish, leafy greens, seeds, and citrus to your grocery list. Grab a high-quality D3 supplement if you're sun deprived. Incorporate magnesium-rich foods or a glycinate supplement before bed.

Throw in a handful of berries and dark chocolate for bonus antioxidant points.

## ☑ Clinical Cues

### ▪ 25-Hydroxyvitamin D [25(OH)D]

Vitamin D can be confusing because the lab range is wide and many women sit at the low end without realizing how much it affects their mood, sleep, and inflammation. Use this cheat sheet to understand where your numbers land and what to ask your provider.

- Normal: 30–100 ng/mL
- Optimal: 50–70 ng/mL

**Why it matters:** Vitamin D acts like a hormone. Low levels are tied to depression, autoimmune flare-ups, and infertility. Women in perimenopause with low D are more likely to have sleep disruption, hot flashes, and bone loss. It also modulates serotonin, explaining why "winter blues" is biochemistry.

### ▪ Ferritin (iron stores)

- Normal: 12–150 ng/mL (women)
- Optimal: 50–100 ng/mL

**Why it matters:** Too low = fatigue, anxiety, restless legs, hair loss. Too high (post-fifty in particular) = inflammation, oxidative stress, increased depression risk. Ferritin is a mood gatekeeper: Women with low stores often describe feeling "wired but tired" and more prone to panic.

## GGT (Gamma-Glutamyl Transferase)

- Normal: 9–38 U/L
- Optimal: <20 U/L

Why it matters: GGT is the oxidative stress marker hiding in plain sight on your basic metabolic panel. Most providers glance at it for liver problems and move on, but GGT is one of the most sensitive early indicators of glutathione depletion, which is your body's master antioxidant and your brain's primary defense against free radical damage. When GGT creeps above 20 U/L, your antioxidant reserves are thinning before anything else looks abnormal. Women dealing with chronic stress, poor sleep, alcohol use, oral contraceptives, or processed food-heavy diets often sit in the 25-45 U/L range, technically "normal," functionally inflamed. Elevated GGT is associated with depression, anxiety, cognitive decline, and increased neuroinflammation. It's also tied to insulin resistance and metabolic dysfunction. The good part? You probably already have this number sitting in old lab work that nobody flagged. Go look. If it's above 20, your brain's antioxidant defense system is running a deficit, and that's oxidative stress doing exactly what we talked about earlier in this chapter.

### RBC Magnesium

- Normal: 4.2–6.8 mg/dL
- Optimal: 5.5–6.5 mg/dL (upper half of range)

**Why it matters:** Magnesium is a cofactor for serotonin and GABA. Stress, alcohol, and oral contraceptives all deplete it. In women, low magnesium = anxiety, PMS cramps, insomnia, and migraines.

### Serum Zinc

- Normal: 60–120 µg/dL
- Optimal: 90–110 µg/dL

**Why it matters:** Zinc balances GABA and glutamate, two neurotransmitters that regulate calm versus wired states. Deficiency = higher risk of postpartum depression and "treatment-resistant" mood disorders.

### Uric Acid

- Normal: 2.5–6.0 mg/dL
- Optimal: 3.5–5.5 mg/dL

**Why it matters:** Uric acid is a Goldilocks marker. Too high and it drives inflammation, oxidative damage, and insulin resistance. Too low and it means your body has lost one of its most abundant natural antioxidants. Most people only hear about uric acid in the context of gout, but in the brain it plays a dual role that directly affects mood and cognition. At optimal levels, uric acid acts as a powerful antioxidant, scavenging free radicals and protecting neurons from oxidative damage. When it climbs above 5.5 mg/dL, it flips from protector to provocateur, triggering inflammatory pathways, raising blood pressure, worsening insulin resistance, and increasing depression and anxiety risk. Women tend to run lower than men thanks to estrogen's uricosuric effect, but that protection fades in perimenopause, which is when uric acid often creeps up alongside mood instability, metabolic shifts, and fatigue that "came out of nowhere." On the other end, uric acid below 3.5 mg/dL can signal depleted antioxidant reserves and has been linked to cognitive decline and increased vulnerability to neuroinflammation. If you already have a CMP or metabolic panel in your records, this number is on it. Check both directions.

## ☑ Moving On

You've fortified your brain with essential vitamins, minerals, and antioxidant defenders. It's time to zoom in on something deceptively simple yet wildly disruptive: blood sugar. Chapter 5 breaks down how even small glucose swings can hijack your mood, spike your anxiety, and leave your focus in shambles. Your brain is not high maintenance; it's just particular. And if you've ever felt hangry, spaced out, or like your nerves were about to stage a walkout, buckle up. This next part is going to make a lot of things click.

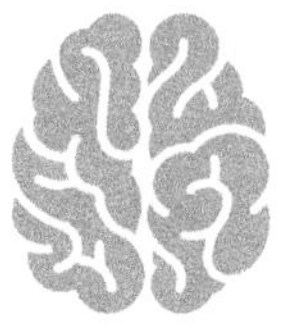



# SUGAR HIGHS, SUGAR LOWS, AND THE EMOTIONAL ROLLER COASTER YOU DIDN'T BUY TICKETS FOR

B lood sugar is non-negotiable fuel for your brain. When it drops too fast or spikes too high, you lose access to the pre-frontal cortex, the part that keeps you reasonable. What's left is pure emotional reactivity and the attention span of a goldfish. We tend to think about blood sugar only in the context of diabetes. Even subtle swings in glucose can whip your mood, focus, and anxiety levels around like you're on the world's worst carnival ride.

Your brain runs almost entirely on glucose. It doesn't store much of it, so it's constantly holding out its hand like "More, please." Give it a balanced, steady stream, and it hums along—calm, focused, emotionally steady. Flood the system with hyperglycemia, and you get a quick dopamine surge, a spike in insulin, and then the inevitable crash: irritability, brain fog, and that "why am I sobbing in the bathroom at work?" feeling.

Let it drop too low (hypoglycemia), and your survival systems kick in. Cue cortisol and adrenaline, stress hormones that, while great for running from bears, are absolute chaos for a modern Wednesday afternoon. You might feel your heart race, palms sweat, head spin, and thoughts spiral into catastrophe, which is exactly why blood sugar dysregulation is a sneaky trigger for anxiety disorders.

I once skipped lunch, drank an iced oat milk latte, and then snapped at my partner over something completely insignificant. Blood sugar isn't just a physical thing; it gets emotional fast.

## The Science Behind the Mood Swings

Blood sugar swings cause more than just a bad mood; they trigger a whole-body biochemical chain reaction. When glucose levels spike quickly, insulin is released to pull sugar into your cells. That's good in theory. This response works well with gradual increases. Sharp spikes, however, trigger insulin overshoot. This drop signals to your brain that fuel is running low, and fast.

Your brain, ever the power-hungry executive, interprets this as a full-blown emergency. In response, your adrenal glands pump out cortisol and adrenaline to raise your blood sugar back up.

These stress hormones evolved for fight-or-flight situations—running from predators, not handling skipped lunches and chocolate bars. The result? You get a chemical cocktail of anxiety, fatigue, shakiness, and mental fog. On a neurotransmitter level, these blood sugar swings interfere with serotonin (your mood stabilizer) and GABA (your calm-and-steady signal), while increasing inflammatory cytokines and oxidative stress. Translation: You feel panicky, moody, exhausted, and wired all at once.

Studies in *Diabetologia* and *The American Journal of Clinical Nutrition* have repeatedly shown that glycemic variability—not just high sugar levels, but frequent swings—is associated with depression, irritability, and anxiety. It's not just what you eat; it's how dramatically your body reacts to it.

And here's a bonus chaos layer: Blood sugar crashes can make PMS symptoms worse. Estrogen and progesterone naturally affect insulin sensitivity throughout your cycle, so if you're already dealing with mood swings, cravings, or irritability, unstable glucose can amplify the noise. Keeping blood sugar steady stabilizes brain function and has documented effects on hormonal signaling, a prescription-free lever.

Functional medicine zooms in tighter than conventional labs. Your doctor might call a fasting glucose of 99 mg/dL "normal," but for brain health, we aim for 75 to 85 mg/dL because that's where energy, focus, and mood tend to stay stable. Fasting insulin under 5 µIU/mL means your cells are responding well to insulin instead of pushing against it.

HbA1c tells you your *average* blood sugar over the past three months. It measures how much glucose has attached itself to your red blood cells as they circulate. Since those cells live about ninety days, HbA1c works like a long-term report card rather than a single-moment snapshot. Ideally it lands between 4.8 and 5.2 percent, which reflects healthy long-term blood sugar control.

This matters because even "high-normal" blood sugar can stress neurons, disrupt neurotransmitter production, and keep your mood stuck on a roller coaster.

## Practical Blood Sugar Zen

The fix isn't complicated, but it does require consistency. The goal: Keep your glucose curve as boring as possible—smooth, gentle rises and falls, no steep climbs or nosedives.

- Start your day with protein and fat instead of just carbs. Think eggs and avocado, not a bagel and regret.
- Pair carbs with protein and fiber. Sweet potato with salmon, apple with almond butter.
- Eat every three to four hours if you're prone to crashes.
- Limit liquid sugar bombs. Soda, juice, and those "healthy" smoothies with 60 g of sugar are emotional land mines.
- Walk after meals. Even ten minutes can blunt a glucose spike and smooth your energy curve.

If you're curious about how your body responds to various foods, a continuous glucose monitor (CGM) can offer real-time feedback. CGMs serve diabetics and nondiabetics alike. Many high-functioning women use them. You can use CGMs for two weeks as a data experiment to figure out which meals or habits send their blood sugar into a tailspin. It's not always what you think.

Also worth noting: Not all sugars behave the same. Glucose is your brain's go-to fuel, while fructose, found in fruit juices and processed sweeteners like high-fructose corn syrup, is metabolized in the liver and doesn't directly feed the brain. Too much fructose can lead to metabolic overload, insulin resistance, and long-term inflammation. So yes, that "natural" juice cleanse may not be doing your mood any favors.

These are simple habits, but they create serious stability for your mood, your brain function, and your overall resilience.

## Bottom Line

Your brain is particular. She needs fuel on schedule, in the right form, and without the chaos of blood sugar spikes and crashes. Balanced blood sugar means fewer anxiety spikes, steadier moods, and a nervous system that isn't white-knuckling through the day. You don't have to go keto, count every gram, or turn meals into math homework. Just aim for balanced meals, strategic snacks, and a glucose curve so uneventful it's almost boring, because boring blood sugar equals a brain that's ready to do epic things.

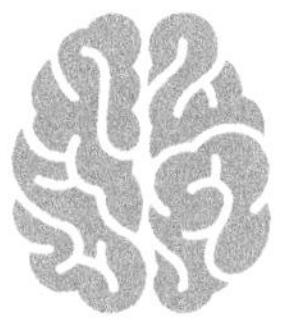



# TL;DR, DO THIS NOW, AND CLINICAL CUES

## ☑ TL;DR

Your brain runs almost exclusively on glucose, but she's not into drama. Big blood sugar swings, either too high or too low, can spike cortisol, scramble neurotransmitters like serotonin and GABA, and leave you anxious, foggy, and emotionally volatile. These fluctuations don't just mess with your mood; they create inflammation, increase oxidative stress, and can even worsen PMS. The goal isn't perfection; it's a smooth, boring glucose curve that lets your nervous system chill out and do its job.

## ☑ Do This Now

- Balance your meals: Every plate should include protein, healthy fats, and fiber. Ditch the naked carbs (looking at you, bagel with nothing on it).

- Time your meals: Eat every three to four hours if you're prone to crashes, and don't skip breakfast unless you're trying to set your mood on fire.

- Watch your drinks: Skip the liquid sugar bombs. Smoothies, juices, and lattes with 45 grams of sugar are not mood friendly.

- Move after eating: A ten-minute walk after meals helps blunt glucose spikes and smooth out your energy.

- Track your patterns: If you're curious or symptomatic, try a continuous glucose monitor (CGM), a wearable sensor that tracks your blood sugar in real time for two weeks, or keep a food + mood journal. Look for emotional dips one to two hours after eating.

- Get curious, not controlling: You don't need to count every carb. You just need to eat in a way that keeps your brain from panicking.

## ☑ Clinical Cues

### ▨ Fasting Glucose

- Normal: 70–99 mg/dL
- Optimal: 75–85 mg/dL

**Why it matters:** High-normal glucose = "I'm fine" fatigue, anxiety flares, worse PMS. Women often get brushed off here, but brains are exquisitely sensitive to even small swings.

### Fasting Insulin

- Normal: 2–25 µIU/mL
- Optimal: <5 µIU/mL

**Why it matters:** Insulin resistance can show up as stubborn weight gain, PCOS, anxiety, and that wired-tired crash after meals.

### HbA1c

- Normal: <5.7%
- Optimal: 4.8–5.2%

**Why it matters:** Reflects three-month blood sugar average. "High-normal" A1c correlates with cognitive decline and mood instability long before diabetes.

### Adiponectin (serum)

**Why it matters:** Anti-inflammatory hormone from fat cells. Higher is better. Low adiponectin signals insulin resistance, chronic inflammation, and unstable brain fuel delivery. Women with low levels often feel puffy, emotionally flat, and metabolically stuck. It drops with poor sleep, sugar, and inactivity. It rises with movement, omega-3s, and Mediterranean-style eating.

### ▪ Lactate (serum, often overlooked outside ICU)

**Why it matters:** Chronically elevated lactate can reflect poor mitochondrial function. Shows up in women as fatigue, exercise intolerance, and brain fog.

### ▪ Leptin (serum)

**Why it matters:** Your brain's "I'm full" signal. High leptin with persistent hunger means leptin resistance: the signal is there but your brain stopped listening. Low leptin (below 4) shows up in under-eating and overtraining, linked to anxiety, insomnia, and lost periods. Leptin resistance also disrupts thyroid, cortisol, and reproductive hormone signaling because the hypothalamus runs all of it. Poor sleep and blood sugar chaos make it worse.

## ☑ Moving On

Once your blood sugar is steady and your energy isn't crashing every three hours, it's time to dig deeper, literally. Because your mood, motivation, and even your sleep might not just depend on what you eat, but what your gut bacteria do with it. In Chapter 6, we'll explore the wild, weird, and wonderful relationship between your belly and your brain. It's not just a connection; it's a full-on biochemical love story.

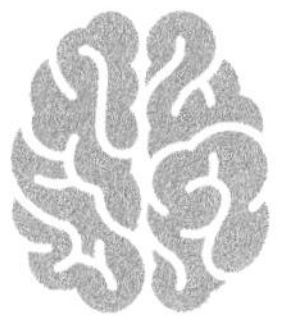



# CHAPTER 6

# THE GUT–BRAIN AXIS: A TALE OF TWO SYSTEMS

The idea that what we eat affects how we feel isn't just a catchy wellness tagline; it's scientific fact, grounded in one of the body's most fascinating communication systems: the gut–brain axis.

This two-way network connects your gastrointestinal (GI) tract with your central nervous system (CNS), allowing constant biochemical dialogue between your belly and your brain. Think of it as a long-distance relationship with excellent communication skills. Your brain and gut are texting, FaceTiming, and occasionally sending each other frantic all-caps messages and voice notes via the vagus nerve.

Here's how what your gut microbes do with what you eat determines how you feel.

## Microbe Town: Where Mood Is Made

Picture your gut as a bustling little village called Microbe Town. It's funky, weird, and filled with bacterial workaholics wearing tiny lab coats. Each species has its own role: Some digest, some defend, and some are elite mood alchemists. Their currency?

The nutrients you send down three times a day.

Let's say you just ate a lentil and sweet potato bowl with a side of kimchi. (Excellent choice.) As that meal travels into Microbe Town, it gets broken down into raw materials: fiber, resistant starches, polyphenols, amino acids, and fermented magic.

Now the real party begins:

- *Lactobacillus,* your GABA specialist, grabs glutamate (from the lentils) and converts it into GABA, your brain's calming neurotransmitter.
- *Escherichia* species (including the friendly kind of *E. coli*) scoop up tryptophan and convert it into serotonin, the original happy hormone that stabilizes your mood and supports sleep.
- Overachieving *E. coli* cousins work with phenylalanine and tyrosine to make dopamine and norepinephrine, your motivation and alertness crew.

But these neurotransmitters don't just hang out in the gut like awkward introverts. They hop onto the vagus nerve, your gut's personal assistant, and head straight to the brain. Think of it as a ten-lane biochemical expressway delivering real-time updates like "Mood's good. Keep the serotonin flowing."

## The Science Behind the Story

Gut bacteria like *Lactobacillus* and *Escherichia* work as biochemical baristas and brain chemists, far more than passive tenants. They help manufacture:

- GABA, to calm your nervous system
- Serotonin, to stabilize mood and support sleep
- Dopamine, for motivation and pleasure
- Norepinephrine, for energy and focus

These molecules either act locally in your gut's own nervous system (yep, your gut has one, called the enteric nervous system, a.k.a. the "second brain"), or they communicate directly with the central nervous system via neural, hormonal, or immune channels.

If the gut–brain axis were a corporate office:

- Your microbiota would be the interns doing 90 percent of the work.
- The vagus nerve would be HR, running interference.
- And your brain would be the moody CEO making all the final calls based on what's coming up from downstairs.

**Quick PSA:** If you've ever taken antibiotics, hormonal birth control, or acid reducers, your microbiome might still be in recovery mode. These meds can deplete beneficial bacteria, which makes feeding your gut the right foods even more important.

## Nourish Your Gut; Fuel Your Mind

The link between gut health and mental wellness has moved from fringe opinion to foundational fact. Studies have connected gut microbiota composition to mood disorders, neurodevelopmental issues, and even neurodegenerative diseases. Probiotics help, but the real work is feeding the system that feeds your brain.

Bonus intel: About 70 percent of your immune system lives in your gut. When your microbiome is thriving, your immune responses are smarter and more stable, which means less inflammation and fewer mood-dampening immune flares.

The powerful part? You control the menu. Every bite is a memo to your microbes. Feed them junk, and chaos follows. Feed them well, and you get calm, clarity, motivation, and better sleep in return.

Some probiotics are now classified as psychobiotics: strains specifically shown to support mood and reduce stress-related symptoms. Think of them as gut bugs with a neuroscience degree. While food should be your foundation, psychobiotics may offer extra support, especially during burnout or recovery.

Personal side note: I didn't think sauerkraut would help my anxiety either. And yet, here we are: me, my nervous system, and my fermented cabbage, thriving.

The old saying holds, you are what you eat. The neuroscience version? You feel what your gut does with what you eat.

Treat your microbiome like the mental health ally it is, and it'll show up for you in ways your multivitamin never could.

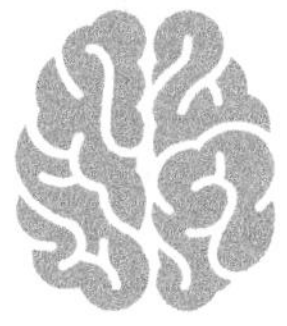



# TL;DR, DO THIS NOW, AND CLINICAL CUES

## ☑ TL;DR

Your gut and your brain are in constant conversation; think of them as biochemical besties. Your gut microbes help produce key neurotransmitters like serotonin, dopamine, GABA, and norepinephrine. But they need the right raw materials: fiber, fermented foods, polyphenols, and prebiotics. When your gut is well fed and balanced, your brain gets calmer, clearer, and more resilient. When it's off? Mood crashes, anxiety spikes, and brain fog come knocking.

## ☑ Do This Now:

- Add one fermented food a day (kimchi, sauerkraut, kefir, plain yogurt).
- Add one prebiotic food a day (garlic, onions, asparagus, bananas, oats).
- Cut one ultra-processed food you rely on (swap protein bars for nuts, cereal for oatmeal).
- Slow down when you eat (put your fork down between bites, chew thoroughly).

## ☑ Clinical Cues

### ▨ High-Sensitivity C-Reactive Protein (hs-CRP)

- Normal: <3 mg/L
- Optimal: <1 mg/L

**Why it matters:** Elevated CRP signals systemic inflammation, which often starts in the gut. Women with bloating, brain fog, or PMS mood swings frequently have hidden low-grade inflammation driving it all. A high CRP in your thirties to fifties can also be an early risk marker for anxiety and depression.

### ▨ Comprehensive Stool Analysis (functional labs like GI-MAP, Genova, etc.)

- Markers: microbiome diversity, short-chain fatty acids, pathogens, yeast, calprotectin

**Why it matters:** More than 90 percent of serotonin is made in the gut. Low microbial diversity = low serotonin resilience → more irritability, low mood, and even PMDD symptoms. A stool test can show if your gut bugs are your hype squad or your saboteurs.

## Zonulin

**Why it matters:** Elevated zonulin = "leaky gut," meaning inflammatory compounds sneak into circulation and spark mood-altering inflammation. Women often feel this as brain fog, food-triggered anxiety, or worsening PMS.

## Vitamin B12 and Folate (serum + functional markers like MMA and homocysteine)

**Why it matters:** Gut health dictates nutrient absorption. If your microbiome is wrecked (antibiotics, birth control, stress), you'll see B-vitamin deficiencies that worsen anxiety, fatigue, and hormonal chaos.

## ☑ Moving On

Now that you know your gut is basically your emotional copilot, it's time to talk food—like, actual meals. Chapter 7 dives into two competing dietary styles: the Mediterranean diet and the ultra-processed Western free-for-all. Spoiler alert: Your brain has a clear favorite. Let's find out which one it is and why your next grocery list might be the most important mental health tool you've got.

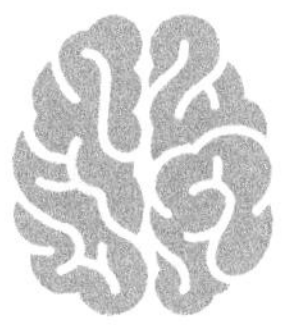



# A FORK IN THE ROAD: MEDITERRANEAN VERSUS WESTERN DIET

Let's say it louder for the burned-out, overwhelmed, anxious girlies in the back: You are what you eat! In a full-body, brain-altering, mood-shifting, thought-clarifying way, not just clearer skin.

Food is chemistry. It's language. Every bite sends a message to your brain, and that message can sound like a lullaby or a chaotic garage band on fire. In her book *This Is Your Brain on Food*, psychiatrist Dr. Uma Naidoo lays it out plain and powerful: The gut–brain axis is real, and our modern diet is trashing our mental health. She's one of many researchers sounding the alarm: What's on your plate shapes your thoughts, regulates your emotions, and determines whether your nervous system supports or sabotages you with poor decision making.

When it comes to long-term mental health, the Mediterranean and Western diets pull you in completely different directions. One nourishes your brain. The other fries it. Let's walk through both.

## The Mediterranean Diet: Food as Medicine

This isn't about sipping wine on a yacht in Santorini (although . . . yes, please). The Mediterranean diet is a centuries-old eating pattern centered around plants, healthy fats, whole grains, and lean proteins, especially fish. It has repeatedly been shown to support everything from heart health to hormone balance, but it also happens to be one of the most powerful dietary approaches for protecting your brain.

Why? Because this way of eating:

- Is rich in anti-inflammatory compounds like omega-3 fatty acids, polyphenols, and antioxidants
- Delivers key nutrients your brain needs (magnesium, B vitamins, folate, zinc)
- Stabilizes blood sugar and supports healthy estrogen metabolism
- Feeds the gut microbiome, which manufactures mood-regulating neurotransmitters like serotonin and GABA
- Reduces oxidative stress and systemic inflammation

The Mediterranean diet actively fertilizes the garden where your calm and clarity grow. That's the loop we want.

I didn't realize how much my diet was wrecking my brain until I was in beautiful Nafplio, Greece, sitting with my family and eating food that tasted alive. By day three of real meals—fresh fish, veggies, olive oil that practically glowed—I could feel my brain being fed, being woken up, almost. A 2022 review in *Nutrients* found that individuals who stuck to a Mediterranean-style diet had significantly lower odds of experiencing depression. Another study in *Molecular Psychiatry* showed a 33 percent reduced risk of depressive symptoms for consistent eaters.

This isn't placebo. This is biology working better.

And here's the beautiful part: It's abundant, delicious, and focused on nourishment instead of restriction. So, let's make it real.

---

## Recipe Break: Your Brain on Greek Salad

*Serves two-to-three crush-worthy humans*

- 1 cucumber, chopped
- 1 cup cherry tomatoes, halved
- ½ red onion, thinly sliced
- ½ cup kalamata olives, pitted
- ¼ cup crumbled feta
- 2 tbsp extra-virgin olive oil
- Juice of 1 lemon
- 1 tsp dried oregano
- Sea salt and black pepper to taste

Toss together. Taste. Adjust. Devour. Bonus points for topping with grilled salmon or chickpeas for protein and a dopamine hit.

## The Western Diet: A Mental Health Dumpster Fire

Look, convenience is queen. We've all had nights when the drive-thru was easier than adulting. But let's call it: The Western diet—ultra-processed foods, added sugars, refined carbs, industrial seed oils—is a public health crisis disguised as self-care.

This is about systems. The Western diet is cheap, addictive, and engineered to hijack your dopamine system. And when you're exhausted, overworked, and running on empty, those hot fries feel like therapy.

The catch? That comfort food is gaslighting your nervous system. It floods your brain with dopamine, spikes your blood sugar, and then leaves you depleted, inflamed, and anxious. It starves your brain of nutrients and actively attacks it.

A 2019 study in *Psychiatry Research* found a clear link between Western diets and depressive symptoms. A 2021 paper in *Frontiers in Psychology* found this style of eating contributes to systemic inflammation that disrupts mood regulation and cognitive clarity.

Ultra-processed foods are engineered to be irresistible. They rewire your brain, train your taste buds, and leave you craving more. Your cravings reflect biochemistry working exactly as designed. Craving is directly related to dopamine. Dopamine is released when you even anticipate a reward, not just when you get one. That little surge pushes you toward the thing that feels exciting, comforting, or satisfying.

## Bottom Line: Choose Your Brain's Adventure

The Mediterranean diet is a daily love letter to your neurons. It's abundant, nourishing, and backed by decades of data showing it protects cognition, balances mood, and supports your stress response.

The Western diet, on the other hand, is a dopamine-depleting cycle of brain fog, burnout, and Sunday scaries. You get to decide: Do you want to feed your brain resilience and clarity, or drip-feed it sabotage dressed in sprinkles?

## A Little Compassion, Because You're Doing Your Best

Aim for function, not perfection. Know what your brain needs, then deliver.

Picture this: You're about to go on a hiking date with the emotionally available cutie from your coworking space. You want to feel good. Light. Present. Capable of walking uphill without dramatic gasping.

The fridge offers two options:

- A leftover breakfast burrito the size of your forearm
- A crisp green bowl piled with arugula, avocado, olive oil, lemon, and a handful of chickpeas or grilled chicken

You know which choice will support your clarity, comfort, and flirting stamina. Skip the guilt. This is about setting yourself up to win, on dates, at work, or just on a random Tuesday when your brain needs a break from the chaos.

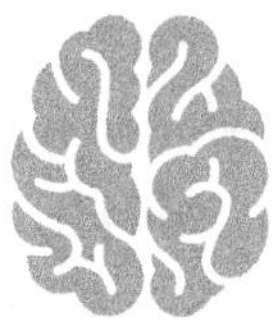



# TL;DR, DO THIS NOW, AND CLINICAL CUES

## ☑ TL;DR

Mediterranean diet = mood magic
Western diet = brain burnout

## ☑ Do This Now

- Add one Mediterranean-style meal this week (Greek salad counts!).
- Swap ultra-processed snacks for nuts, fruit, or hummus and veggies.
- Cook with olive oil instead of seed oils.

- Try eating more legumes, leafy greens, fatty fish, and fermented foods.
- Don't aim for perfection; aim for progress that supports your brain.

## ☑ Clinical Cues

### ▣ Lipid Panel (total cholesterol, LDL, HDL, triglycerides)

- Normal: TC <200 mg/dL, LDL <100, HDL >40 (women ideally >50), triglycerides <150
- Optimal: LDL <100, HDL >60, triglycerides <100

**Why it matters:** Western diets drive triglycerides up and HDL down, which worsens inflammation and brain perfusion. Mediterranean patterns raise HDL (the "cleanup crew") and lower triglycerides, directly improving mood stability and cognitive health.

### ▣ Omega-3 Index (EPA and DHA % of total fatty acids)

- Normal: ≥4%
- Optimal: 8–12%

**Why it matters:** Mediterranean diets supply abundant omega-3s from fish, nuts, and olive oil, buffering mood and protecting against depression. Western diets loaded with seed oils and processed fats suppress this marker.

■ **High-Sensitivity C-Reactive Protein (hs-CRP)**

- Normal: <3 mg/L
- Optimal: <1 mg/L

**Why it matters:** Western diets elevate CRP through refined carbs and industrial oils, creating systemic inflammation. Mediterranean eating lowers CRP, translating into calmer moods, less anxiety, and better hormone balance.

■ **Fasting Glucose and Insulin**

- Normal: glucose 70–99 mg/dL, insulin 2–25 µIU/mL
- Optimal: glucose 75–85 mg/dL, insulin <5 µIU/mL

**Why it matters:** Western-style eating promotes insulin resistance, which manifests in women as fatigue, PMS mood crashes, and perimenopausal weight gain. Mediterranean eating improves insulin sensitivity and stabilizes brain fuel supply.

## ☑ Moving On

So you've fed your brain the good stuff. Now what about the supplements that claim to "biohack" your focus and mood? In the next chapter, we're entering the wild west of wellness; nootropics and adaptogens. Some are legit. Some are snake oil, and we're going to learn how to tell the difference. Let's go.

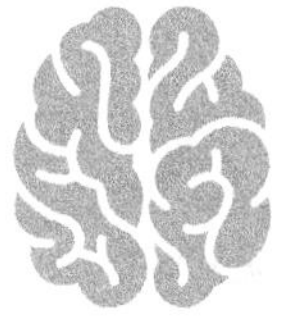



# SMART DRUGS AND STRESS PLANTS: A SKEPTICAL LOVE LETTER TO NOOTROPICS AND ADAPTOGENS

Welcome to the part of the wellness aisle, where things get weird. On one side: powdered mushrooms with names like lion's mane and reishi, promising to "nourish your nervous system." On the other: sleek nootropic stacks with fonts that look like Elon Musk personally approved them, claiming to turn you into a productivity cyborg.

Let's talk about nootropics and adaptogens because you deserve to know which brain-boosting supplements actually work and which are just expensive snake oil.

## Nootropics: The Smart-Drug Myth (But Also Maybe Not?)

Nootropics are substances—natural, synthetic, or somewhere in between—that supposedly enhance cognitive function. Think memory, focus, motivation, and that elusive thing called mental clarity (which, if we're honest, most of us haven't felt since 2016).

Let's start with the legit, science-backed stuff:

- **Caffeine and L-theanine**
  Found in tea, caffeine wakes you up, and L-theanine smooths out the anxiety. It's the millennial anxiety cocktail of choice, and research backs it up. Together, they improve attention and reduce the jittery mess.
  Findings show caffeine plus L-theanine improves attention, mood stability, and reduces anxiety symptoms. [Haskell et al. (2008) *Biological Psychology*]

- **Creatine**
  Creatine works for brains, not just muscles. It helps supply energy to brain cells and has shown cognitive benefits in sleep-deprived people and vegetarians.
  [Rae et al. (2003) *Proceedings of the Royal Society: Biological Sciences*]

- **Citicoline and Alpha-GPC**

  These choline sources support acetylcholine production, a neurotransmitter tied to memory and learning. Research shows small but measurable improvements in cognitive performance, especially in people with mild impairment or sleep deprivation. Promising, but biology moves in inches, not leaps. More high-quality studies needed. [Wignall and Brown (2014); García-Cabrera et al. (2020)]

- *Bacopa monnieri*

  An herb used in Ayurvedic medicine that may improve memory formation and recall, particularly with consistent use over several months. Research shows it can reduce anxiety and improve information processing, though it works slowly; think weeks to months, not days. Generally well tolerated, but can cause digestive upset in some people. [Calabrese et al. (2008) *British Journal of Clinical Pharmacology;* Pase et al. (2012) *Journal of Alternative and Complementary Medicine*]

Then there are the overpromising start-up blends with names like Neurazenx and Quantum Clarity, containing fifty-seven ingredients you can't pronounce. These are often based on shaky evidence, small studies, or "ancient wisdom" repackaged in $80 bottles. And beware of "proprietary blends." It's Latin for "We're not telling you how much of anything is in here."

- **Ginkgo and Ginseng Callout** And then there's ginkgo biloba and ginseng, plastered on everything from energy drinks to brain pills. Ginkgo has been studied extensively for memory and cognitive decline, but results are inconsistent at best. Ginseng (especially panax) shows up everywhere in wellness marketing, with claims about energy and focus, but the evidence is mixed and highly dependent on quality and dosage. Both might help some people, but they're not the cognitive game changers the marketing suggests.

## Reality Check

Most nootropics don't work like a triple shot of espresso. They take time. You're not going to suddenly feel like Bradley Cooper in *Limitless* after two days on L-theanine. These compounds often work cumulatively, supporting neurotransmitter pathways, energy metabolism, or neural resilience over weeks or months.

True story: The first time I tried L-theanine, I half expected to feel like a productivity robot by lunch. Instead, I got a mild headache and forgot where I left my phone. Turns out, it wasn't the miracle I hoped for, but a reminder to eat breakfast first.

And here's a spicy truth: Sometimes the ritual helps as much as the substance itself. The placebo effect is powerful, especially when your nervous system is looking for a reason to believe it's safe. So if your brain relaxes every time you sip your $9 adaptogenic latte? That's still healing. Rituals matter.

## Adaptogens: Ancient Herbs, Modern Stress

Now onto adaptogens: a class of herbs and fungi that allegedly help your body adapt to stress by regulating the HPA axis, the system that controls your stress hormones like cortisol.

They're not new. People have been using these for centuries in Ayurveda and Traditional Chinese Medicine. What's new is the rebrand, the influencer unboxings, and the $39.99 mushroom tinctures with forestcore fonts.

The top contenders:

- **Ashwagandha**
  The chill pill of the herbal world. Research suggests it can reduce cortisol and anxiety in chronically stressed humans. This is nervous system support for people who lose their grip over missing socks, slow-loading apps, or accidentally hitting "Reply All."
  [Chandrasekhar et al. (2012) *Indian Journal of Psychological Medicine*]

- **Rhodiola Rosea**
  May improve fatigue, focus, and stress resilience, especially when you're running on fumes and passive aggression.
  [Panossian and Wikman (2010) *Current Clinical Pharmacology*]

- **Reishi and Lion's Mane**
  Mushrooms that might support immunity, mood, and neurogenesis, meaning your body's ability to grow new

neurons. The evidence is early but interesting, especially for lion's mane, which may support nerve growth factor (NGF) and improve mild cognitive impairment. [Mori et al. (2009) *Biomedical Research*]

- **Cordyceps** A fungus traditionally used to boost energy and athletic performance. Some research suggests it may improve oxygen utilization and reduce fatigue, though most studies are small. Popular in the biohacking crowd, but the evidence is still building. Worth trying if you're curious, but don't expect miracles. [Hirsch et al. (2017) *Journal of Dietary Supplements*]

- **Holy Basil (Tulsi)**
  Traditionally used for everything from anxiety to blood sugar regulation. Jury's still out, but it's generally safe and has some decent preliminary research. [Jamshidi and Cohen (2017) *Evidence-Based Complementary and Alternative Medicine*]

## Gut Check: Supplement Quality Matters

The supplement industry lacks regulation, so quality varies dramatically. The industry isn't well regulated, which means potency and purity can vary wildly. Look for products that are third-party tested (by NSF, USP, or Informed Choice) and brands that list actual dosages, instead of just fairy-dusting a cool-sounding herb over a bunch of filler ingredients.

Bottom line: Some supplements seem to have some pretty cool qualities. But there's no replacement for a life that feels good to you, and there's no point in wasting cash on supplements that are just pricey dust.

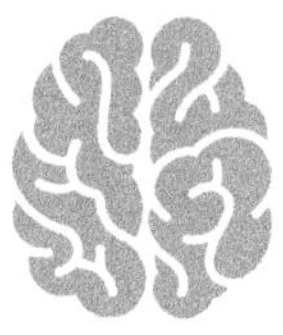



# TL;DR, DO THIS NOW, AND CLINICAL CUES

## ☑ TL;DR

- Nootropics are brain-boosting compounds, some of which have real benefits (like L-theanine, caffeine, and creatine), but most are overhyped.
- Adaptogens like ashwagandha and rhodiola may help regulate stress, especially when used consistently over time.
- Think of supplements as sidekicks, not miracle workers.
- Quality matters. Look for transparency, testing, and actual dosages.
- Ritual matters too. If it calms you, supports a routine, and gives your brain a breather? That's legit, even if it's technically a placebo.

## ☑ Do This Now

- Choose one adaptogen or nootropic that matches your current need (like calm, energy, or focus) and try it for four to six weeks.
- Don't skip the basics: Hydration, food, movement, and rest matter more than any supplement.
- When shopping, skip the mystery blends. Look for transparency and third-party testing.
- Track how you feel, not just physically, but emotionally and cognitively. Subtle shifts count.

## ☑ Clinical Cues

### Cortisol (saliva or serum, ideally four-point diurnal curve)

- Normal a.m.: 6–23 µg/dL with steady decline into evening
- Optimal: 10–18 µg/dL in the morning with a clear curve down to <5 µg/dL at night

**Why it matters:** Adaptogens like ashwagandha, rhodiola, and holy basil fine-tune your cortisol curve. A flat or inverted rhythm (wired at night, wiped in the morning) is common in women aged thirty to sixty with chronic stress, insomnia, or perimenopausal sleep issues.

### ■ DHEA-S

- Reference: ~ 35–430 µg/dL
- Optimal: ~200–350 µg/dL (Age dependent, not appropriate for women over 50.)

**Why it matters:** DHEA is the nervous system''s biological shock absorber. Chronic mental overload, perfectionism, and nonstop "doing mode" drain it. Low DHEA = low resilience: brain fog, depleted motivation, emotional fragility.

### ■ High-Sensitivity C-Reactive Protein (hs-CRP)

- Normal: <3 mg/L
- Optimal: <1 mg/L

**Why it matters:** Adaptogens have anti-inflammatory effects. Elevated CRP suggests chronic stress is inflaming both body and brain, leading to anxiety, irritability, and fatigue.

### ■ Adrenocorticotropic Hormone (ACTH, optional)

**Why it matters:** Paired with cortisol, ACTH can show if the brain is overdriving adrenal output. Helpful for women who feel "burnt out" despite normal one-time cortisol snapshots.

## ☑ Moving On

You've just walked through the biochemical jungle of fats, vitamins, minerals, blood sugar, gut bugs, mood food, and herbal enhancers. You've made it out smarter, sassier, and way more equipped to decode your own brain chemistry.

Before we dive into more advanced strategies, let's take a moment to summarize what we've learned so far, connect the dots, and give your nervous system a hot second to breathe.

Because knowledge without integration is just more noise, and you're not here for noise. You're here to feel good.

Ready to recap? Let's roll into the Part 1 Recap.

# PART 1 RECAP

## Feed Your Brain (Literally)

Every nutrient deficiency you just learned about (low omega-3s, depleted B vitamins, insufficient vitamin D, unstable blood sugar, disrupted gut health) directly drains your nervous system's load capacity.

When your iron is at the low end of "normal," your brain is running on reduced oxygen, burning through capacity just to maintain basic function. When your B12 is suboptimal, neurotransmitter production slows, and suddenly that work email feels insurmountable.

This is why Part 1 matters for your mental health: Every biological deficit you address restores capacity. You're increasing your nervous system's ability to handle life. As you move into your hormones, movement, connection, mindfulness, and hobbies, remember that these interventions work exponentially better when your biological foundation is solid. Feed your brain first; then teach it to regulate.

A quick review of chapters:

## 🧠 Chapter 1: Your Brain Is a Messy, Brilliant Energy Hog

- Your brain is only 2% of your body weight but burns 20% to 25% of your energy.
- Mood swings, brain fog, and anxiety often signal under-fueled brain chemistry rather than fundamental dysfunction.

- You might just be undernourished, overstimulated, and running on fumes.

## 🐟 Chapter 2: The Fatty Acid Trip

- Omega-3s (especially EPA and DHA) are critical for mood, memory, and reducing brain inflammation,
- ALA from plants is good but not enough; you need marine sources or algae-based supplements.
- Aim for 500 to 1,000 mg EPA and DHA daily, and your neurons will throw a gratitude party.

## 💊 Chapter 3: The B-Vitamin Brain Boost

- B6, B12, and folate are your neurotransmitter construction crew.
- Deficiencies can mimic depression, anxiety, PMS, fatigue, and even paranoia.
- Methylated B complexes may be especially helpful if you have the MTHFR gene variant (hi, 40% of the population). Bonus: They help with hormone detox and estrogen balance too.

## ⬡ Chapter 4: The Mineral Squad and Vitamin D

- Low vitamin D is *strongly linked* to depression, seasonal and otherwise.

- Optimal blood levels? Aim for 50 to 70 ng/mL, not just "within range."
- Zinc, magnesium, and iron are foundational for making neurotransmitters.
- Oxidative stress (the inflammation chaos agent) damages brain cells, and antioxidants are your shield.

## ◈ Chapter 5: Sugar, Spikes, and Meltdowns

- Your brain loves glucose, but it likes consistency, not chaos.
- Blood-sugar crashes trigger cortisol and adrenaline, leading to anxiety and emotional spirals.
- Balanced meals (protein, fat, fiber) keep your mood stable and your brain chill.
- Bonus: glucose balance = hormone balance. Yes, even your period symptoms improve.

## 🐥 Chapter 6: Gut Feelings Are Real Feelings

- Your gut and brain are in constant conversation via the vagus nerve.
- Gut microbes help produce GABA, serotonin, dopamine, and more.
- Feeding your microbiome with fiber, fermented foods, and prebiotics supports emotional resilience.
- Antibiotics, birth control, and acid reducers disrupt gut health, but you can rebuild.

- Psychobiotics are probiotics that support mood specifically (and yes, they're a thing).

## 🥗 Chapter 7: Food Is Mood

- The Mediterranean diet feeds your brain, gut, and mitochondria.
- The Western diet feeds inflammation, mood swings, and regret.
- You don't need perfection, just consistency, awareness, and food that actually makes you feel good.
- Bottom line: Food can either regulate your brain or hijack it. You choose.

## 🍄 Chapter 8: Nootropics and Adaptogens

- Some nootropics (caffeine and L-theanine, creatine) are legit. Most are overhyped.
- Adaptogens like ashwagandha and rhodiola support your stress response. They work alongside rest, never as a replacement.
- Supplements can help, but rituals, consistency, and the basics matter more.
- You're still the main character. Supplements are just your supporting cast.

## 💡 Integration Time and Moving On

You now have a full kit of nutritional tools: fats, vitamins, minerals, blood sugar, gut health, whole-food patterns, and supplemental support. You've learned how they connect to your brain chemistry, hormones, energy, and emotions.

The goal? Start with one system at a time.

Maybe you're low on omega-3s.

Maybe your gut is crying out for some fermented food and fiber.

Maybe your mood is screaming, "B12 me!" and you just haven't listened yet.

That's the magic of functional nutrition. It's not about fixing one thing; it's about supporting the whole ecosystem of *you*.

So now you know your brain is basically a bougie chemistry lab. One that runs on leafy greens, stable blood sugar, healthy fats, and the occasional fermented sidekick. The critical variable: Even the best fuel needs an engine that actually runs.

Part 1 gave you the raw materials. Part 2 is where we learn when your body actually wants them. Because your brain doesn't just need the right nutrients. It needs them at the right time, in sync with a hormonal rhythm most of us were never taught to track. Your estrogen, progesterone, cortisol, and insulin aren't just floating around randomly. They're running a tightly choreographed relay, and when one leg falters, your mood, energy, and mental clarity take the hit.

This next section is about learning the language your hormones have been speaking all along: the one that explains why you feel unstoppable one week and completely depleted the next. Get ready to decode your cycle and understand what your labs are telling you at each phase. Let's get into the science your body has been waiting for you to learn.

# PART 2

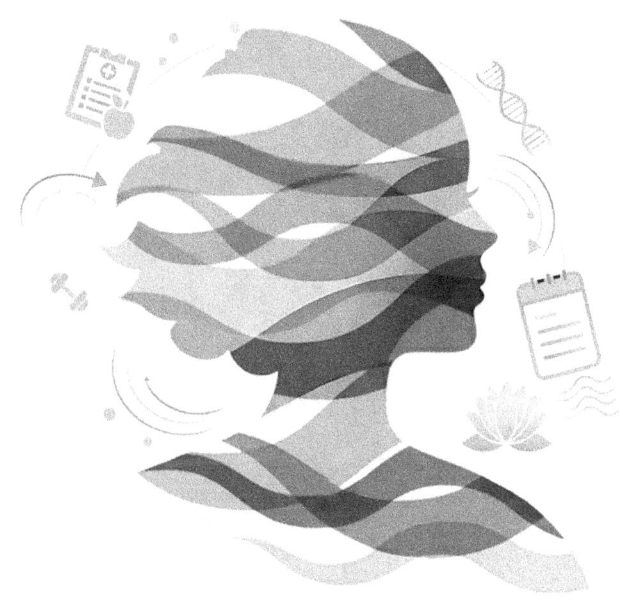

# YOUR HORMONES AND YOUR CYCLE

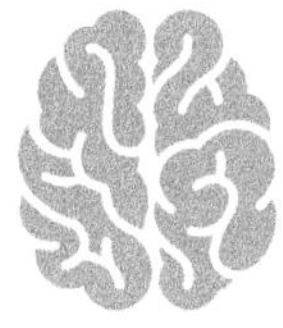



# YOUR CYCLE, PERIMENOPAUSE, MENOPAUSE, AND YOUR BRAIN

Your hormones are the operating system your brain runs on. When they shift, everything shifts with them. This chapter is about understanding those shifts, so you stop blaming yourself for what your biochemistry is doing.

## Your Menstrual Cycle Is a Brain Event

Most of us were taught that our menstrual cycle is about reproduction. Ovulation, periods, fertility. That framing is not wrong, but it is wildly incomplete. Your cycle is a 25- to 35-day orchestration of chemical signals between your hypothalamus, your pituitary gland, and your ovaries, and it directly controls your mood, your energy, your cognition, your sleep architecture, and your stress tolerance.

Every month, your brain chemistry rewrites itself. Not metaphorically. *Literally.* The neurotransmitters that regulate how you feel (serotonin, dopamine, GABA, norepinephrine) are all modulated by estrogen and progesterone. When those hormones shift, your neurochemistry shifts with them. This is the biochemistry.

## The Four Phases

Your cycle has four distinct phases, and each one changes the way your brain operates.

1.  The **menstrual phase** runs roughly from day one through day five. Estrogen and progesterone are both at their lowest point. Serotonin drops. Energy is low. Many women experience brain fog, fatigue, increased pain sensitivity, and low motivation during this phase. Your nervous system is running on the smallest fuel supply of the entire month.
    a.  This is not the time to push through. This is the time to rest, and there is nothing lazy about it.
2.  The **follicular phase** spans approximately day six through day thirteen. Estrogen begins climbing, and it brings dopamine and serotonin up with it. You start to feel sharper.

More creative. More social. Your working memory improves. Your verbal fluency increases.

a.   This is when your brain is primed for new projects, hard conversations, strategic thinking, and problem solving. If you have ever noticed that some weeks you feel unstoppable and other weeks you can barely deal with your coworkers, this is why.

3.   The **ovulatory phase** is the shortest, lasting roughly day fourteen through day sixteen. Estrogen peaks. Testosterone surges briefly. Luteinizing hormone triggers egg release.

a.   This is when most women report feeling the most confident, the most energized, and the most like the version of themselves they wish they could be all the time. That version is not an imaginary sense of self. She is a reflection of your hormones at their highest point.

4.   The **luteal phase** runs from approximately day seventeen through day twenty-eight. Progesterone rises while estrogen drops. Progesterone is supposed to have a calming effect through its action on GABA receptors. But if your progesterone is insufficient, or if the ratio between progesterone and estrogen is off, you get anxiety instead of calm. Insomnia instead of deep sleep. Irritability, cravings, bloating, and mood swings.

a.   This is where PMS lives. This is also where PMDD lives. And this is the phase most often dismissed as you just being emotional. If you feel like a completely different person in the second half of your cycle, that's biology. That is a progesterone to estrogen ratio that your labs can quantify.

## What Your Labs Should Include During Your Cycling Years

Timing matters when you are still cycling. Baseline hormones should be drawn on day three of your cycle. Progesterone should be drawn on day twenty-one to confirm ovulation and assess luteal function. A single random draw will miss the picture.

Start with estradiol, which is your primary estrogen and the main driver of follicular phase energy and mood. Low estradiol on day three may signal declining ovarian reserve or suppression from chronic stress. Progesterone on day twenty-one confirms whether you actually ovulated and whether your luteal phase has enough hormonal support. Low progesterone is one of the most common and most overlooked causes of anxiety, insomnia, and short cycles.

FSH, or follicle stimulating hormone, tells you how hard your brain is working to get your ovaries to respond. When FSH starts rising on day three, it means the ovaries are losing sensitivity. This is one of the earliest flags for perimenopause, and it can show up years before your cycle changes.

LH, or luteinizing hormone, triggers ovulation. The ratio of LH to FSH matters. Elevated LH with relatively low FSH can point toward a PCOS pattern.

Total and free testosterone drive libido, motivation, and muscle tone. Too high suggests androgen excess. Too low and you get fatigue, flat mood, and low drive. DHEA-S is your adrenal androgen precursor, and low levels often correlate with what gets called adrenal fatigue. SHBG, or sex hormone binding globulin, controls how much of your sex hormones are actually bioavailable. Low SHBG means more free testosterone circulating, which can show up as acne and hair loss. High SHBG means less bioavailable estrogen, even if your total estrogen looks fine on paper.

Your thyroid panel should include TSH, free T3, free T4, and TPO antibodies. Not just TSH alone. Subclinical hypothyroidism mimics depression, causes irregular cycles, and gets missed constantly when only TSH is tested. Morning cortisol or a 4-point salivary cortisol panel reveals your stress hormone pattern. Chronic cortisol elevation steals pregnenolone away from progesterone production, which means the more stressed you are, the less progesterone you make.

Fasting insulin and glucose give you a metabolic baseline. Insulin resistance disrupts ovulation and increases androgen production, creating a vicious cycle. Vitamin D is a hormone precursor and immune modulator, and deficiency is linked to worse PMS, mood disorders, and autoimmune flares. Ferritin is your iron storage marker, and it is not the same as serum iron.

Below 50 ng/mL and you will experience fatigue, hair loss, and brain fog even if your hemoglobin is completely normal. B12 and folate are essential for methylation and neurotransmitter synthesis. When they are low, your body cannot efficiently produce serotonin or dopamine.

## Perimenopause: The Transition Nobody Warned You About

Perimenopause is not a switch that flips. It is a slow, erratic process that can begin as early as your mid-thirties and last anywhere from four to ten years before your final period. Most women are not told this is happening. Most doctors are not testing for it. And most of the symptoms get attributed to stress, aging, or anxiety disorders.

Here is what is actually happening. Your ovaries start producing estrogen and progesterone erratically. Some months you overproduce estrogen. Some months you barely make any progesterone. The ratio between the two, the ratio your brain has relied on for decades to regulate mood, sleep, and cognition, becomes unreliable. And your nervous system responds accordingly.

## What Perimenopause Looks Like

Anxiety that shows up out of nowhere, sometimes as a physical sensation in your chest before it ever becomes a thought. Insomnia that does not respond to melatonin or sleep hygiene. Rage that feels disproportionate to the situation. Brain fog so thick you forget words mid-sentence. Heart palpitations that send you to the ER only to be told your heart is fine. Migraines that change pattern or appear for the first time. Joint pain. New histamine reactions. Weight gain concentrated around your midsection despite no changes in diet or exercise. Cycles that get shorter, then longer, then skip entirely. And when you go to the doctor, your labs come back normal.

Normal does not mean optimal. A TSH of 4.2 is in range. It is not where your brain functions well. An estradiol of 40 pg/mL is "normal for your age." It may also be the reason you cannot sleep.

The problem with testing in perimenopause is that hormone levels fluctuate wildly from week to week. A single snapshot can miss the entire picture. This is why I recommend testing on day three when possible and tracking trends over three to six months rather than relying on a single draw.

A DUTCH test, which stands for Dried Urine Test for Comprehensive Hormones, provides metabolite level detail that serum testing alone cannot capture. It shows you not just how much estrogen you are producing, but how your body is processing and clearing it, which matters enormously for both symptom management and long-term risk.

## What to Test in Perimenopause

Everything from your cycling years panel still applies, but with added context. Estradiol will be fluctuating wildly. A single normal result does not rule out perimenopause. You need the trend. Progesterone, drawn at day twenty-one, is often the first hormone to decline meaningfully. When progesterone drops but estrogen stays intact or spikes, you end up in a state of relative estrogen dominance. That pattern drives anxiety, heavy periods, fibroid growth, and breast tenderness.

FSH on day three above 25 mIU/mL is a strong signal that your ovaries are losing their responsiveness. AMH, or anti-Mullerian hormone, tracks your ovarian reserve. It is not diagnostic on its own, but it helps map where you are in the transition.

Cortisol testing becomes even more critical during this phase. When your ovaries start declining, your adrenal glands attempt to compensate. If your adrenals are already depleted from years of chronic stress, the transition accelerates and symptoms intensify. A 4-point salivary cortisol or a DUTCH cortisol panel will show you the pattern.

Thyroid dysfunction frequently unmasks during perimenopause. If you have Hashimoto's, expect flares during this transition. Always check TPO antibodies, not just TSH. Fasting insulin, glucose, and HbA1c become more important now because estrogen decline removes a layer of metabolic protection. This is when insulin resistance can take hold, and it is when Type 2 diabetes risk begins climbing.

Add hs-CRP to your panel as an inflammatory marker. Rising systemic inflammation drives the joint pain, brain fog, and cardiovascular risk that accelerate during perimenopause. Homocysteine reflects your methylation efficiency, and elevated levels are both a cardiovascular risk factor and an indicator that your neurotransmitter metabolism is compromised.

Your micronutrient panel matters more now than ever. Vitamin D, magnesium (measured as RBC magnesium, not serum), B12, ferritin, and folate should all be monitored. Deficiencies that your body could compensate for in your twenties become symptomatic much faster as your hormonal buffering decreases. An omega-3 index below 8% is associated with increased risk of depression and cognitive decline, both of which are already elevated during this transition.

## Menopause: The New Baseline

Menopause is defined as twelve consecutive months without a period. The average age is fifty-one, but it can happen earlier or later. The key thing to understand is that menopause is not the start of the shift. The shift started years ago during perimenopause. Menopause is when the new baseline settles in.

After menopause, estrogen drops to a permanently low level. Progesterone is essentially gone. Testosterone continues a gradual decline. And the systems that relied on these hormones for decades, your brain, your bones, your cardiovascular system, your gut, your skin, start showing the cumulative effect.

## What Menopause Looks Like

For some women, the acute symptoms of perimenopause ease. Hot flashes may lessen. The mood swings may calm. But new patterns emerge. Vaginal dryness and urinary changes become common. Bone density begins accelerating its decline. Cardiovascular risk increases significantly, because estrogen was doing more to protect your heart than most women realize.

Cognitive shifts range from mild word finding difficulty to genuine concern about dementia. Mood may settle into a lower, flatter baseline rather than the dramatic swings of perimenopause. Skin thins. Muscle mass decreases. Sleep may never quite return to what it was.

The first five years after menopause are when bone density drops fastest and cardiovascular risk increases most sharply. This is not the time to stop testing. This is the time to test smarter.

## What to Test After Menopause

Cycle timing no longer applies. You can test anytime, but aim for consistency. Same time of day, same conditions. If you are on hormone replacement therapy, test twelve to twenty-four hours after your last dose to capture trough levels.

Estradiol below 20 pg/mL is common post-menopause, but it is also associated with accelerated cognitive decline and cardiovascular risk. Estrone, which is the dominant estrogen after menopause and is primarily made in fat tissue, should be monitored as well. Elevated estrone with low estradiol may indicate poor estrogen metabolism. If you are on HRT, progesterone testing confirms adequate dosing for endometrial protection.

FSH above 40 mIU/mL confirms menopausal status. Total and free testosterone continue to matter because low testosterone drives muscle loss, low libido, and the flat, colorless mood that many post-menopausal women describe.

Your thyroid panel becomes more important, not less. Autoimmune thyroid disease incidence increases after menopause, and Hashimoto's can progress. Monitor both TPO and thyroglobulin antibodies.

Metabolic markers are essential. Fasting insulin, glucose, and HbA1c should be tracked because without estrogen's insulin-sensitizing effect, glucose regulation deteriorates. Request an advanced lipid panel that includes LDL particle number, lipoprotein(a), and ApoB. Standard lipid panels miss the atherogenic particle count that actually predicts cardiovascular events. hs-CRP and homocysteine are both independent cardiovascular risk factors that increase post-menopause. A DEXA scan for bone density paired with a vitamin D level gives you the full picture on skeletal health. Vitamin D below 50 ng/mL impairs calcium absorption and accelerates bone loss. Magnesium RBC reflects your true intracellular magnesium stores, which serum magnesium does not. B12, folate, and ferritin round out your nutrient panel, but note that post-menopausal women can also develop iron overload, so monitoring the upper end of the ferritin range matters just as much as the lower end.

Cortisol testing remains important because after menopause, your adrenal glands are your primary remaining source of hormones. Protecting adrenal function is not optional. It is survival strategy.

## The Real Conversation

None of these transitions are things that happen to you while you sit helplessly by. They are biological events, and biological events can be measured, tracked, supported, and managed. But only if someone is actually looking.

The gap between how you feel and what your labs say is not proof that nothing is wrong. It is proof that the wrong things are being measured, or the right things are being measured against the wrong standards.

You deserve more than a shrug and a prescription for an SSRI when what you actually need is a full hormone panel drawn at the right time in your cycle, a provider who understands the difference between reference ranges and functional ranges, and someone who believes you the first time you say something feels off.

Your body has been trying to tell you. Now you have the science to back it up.

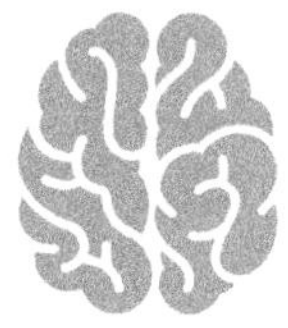

## CHAPTER 9.5

# TL;DR, DO THIS NOW, AND CLINICAL CUES

### ☑ TL;DR

Your menstrual cycle is a monthly neurochemical reset with four phases that directly control your mood, energy, cognition, and stress tolerance. Estrogen and progesterone are not just reproductive hormones. They modulate serotonin, dopamine, and GABA, which means when they shift, your entire mental health landscape shifts with them. Perimenopause can start as early as your mid-30s and last up to a decade, producing anxiety, brain fog, rage, insomnia, and a dozen other symptoms that get dismissed because your labs come back "normal." Menopause settles your hormones at a permanently low baseline, and the systems they were protecting, your brain, your bones, your heart, your metabolism, begin showing the wear. At every phase, the gap between "in range" and "feeling like yourself" is where the real clinical conversation starts.

## ☑ Do This Now

If you are still cycling, schedule labs for day three of your next cycle (baseline hormones) and day twenty-one (progesterone). If you are in perimenopause, get a day three draw and plan to repeat it in three to six months so you can track the trend instead of relying on a single snapshot.

If you are post-menopausal, pick a consistent time of day and get your panel drawn. Request the full list below, not just TSH and a CBC. If your provider pushes back, find one who will run them or order through a direct-to-consumer lab service. Bring this chapter with you to your appointment. Use the Lab Tracker in the back of this book to record every result. A single draw is a photograph. Your health is a movie. Start filming.

## ☑ Clinical Cues

This short guide helps you understand how to read your hormone labs the way a clinician does. "Normal" reflects the broad lab reference interval. "Optimal" shows the range where most women feel and function their best. Use these cues to understand your own results and recognize when a value that is technically fine might still be dragging down your mood, sleep, or energy.

### ▪ Estradiol (E2)

- Normal (follicular): 30 to 120 pg/mL
- Normal (mid-cycle): 100 to 400 pg/mL
- Normal (luteal): 50 to 250 pg/mL
- Optimal: Varies by phase, but mid-follicular above 60 pg/mL and mid-cycle above 150 pg/mL is where most women report stable mood and sharp cognition.

**Why it matters:** Estradiol is the primary estrogen driving your brain's serotonin and dopamine activity. Low estradiol on Day 3 can signal declining ovarian reserve or chronic stress suppression. In perimenopause, levels fluctuate wildly, so a single normal result does not rule anything out. Post-menopause, levels below 20 pg/mL are associated with accelerated cognitive decline and cardiovascular risk.

### ▪ Progesterone (mid-luteal, Day 21)

- Normal: 2–25 ng/mL in the luteal phase
- Optimal: 10 to 25 ng/mL mid-luteal

**Why it matters:** Progesterone is your calming hormone. It acts on GABA receptors to promote sleep, reduce anxiety, and stabilize mood in the second half of your cycle. Low progesterone with intact estrogen creates relative estrogen dominance, which drives PMS, heavy periods, fibroids, breast tenderness, and luteal phase anxiety. In perimenopause, progesterone is usually the first hormone to decline meaningfully. If you are waking at 3 a.m. with a racing heart during your luteal phase, this is the number to check.

### FSH (Follicle Stimulating Hormone)

- Normal (Day 3): 3 to 10 mIU/mL during reproductive years
- Perimenopause flag: Above 25 mIU/mL on Day 3 suggests ovaries are losing responsiveness
- Menopause confirmed: Above 40 mIU/mL consistently

**Why it matters:** FSH is your brain's signal to your ovaries to produce follicles. Rising FSH on day three is one of the earliest indicators that the perimenopausal transition has begun, often years before your cycle visibly changes. If your anxiety or insomnia started "out of nowhere" in your late thirties or forties, FSH is one of the first things to check.

### LH (Luteinizing Hormone)

- Normal (Day 3): 2 to 15 mIU/mL

**Why it matters:** LH triggers ovulation. The ratio of LH to FSH matters more than either number alone. An LH to FSH ratio above 2:1 can suggest a PCOS pattern. In perimenopause, LH rises alongside FSH as the brain works harder to stimulate the ovaries.

### ▦ Testosterone (Total, Female)

- Normal: 15 to 70 ng/dL
- Optimal: 30 to 60 ng/dL

**Why it matters:** Low testosterone shows up as fatigue, low libido, loss of motivation, and flat mood. High testosterone with other androgen markers points toward PCOS. Testosterone continues declining gradually after menopause and contributes to muscle loss and the emotional flatness many women describe.

### ▦ Free Testosterone (Female)

- Normal: 0.1 to 6.4 pg/mL

**Why it matters:** Free testosterone is the amount that is actually bioavailable. Total testosterone can look normal while free testosterone is tanked because SHBG is too high, or free testosterone is elevated because SHBG is too low. This number tells the real story.

### ▦ DHEA-S

- Normal: 35 to 430 mcg/dL (age-dependent, declines over time)
- Optimal: Middle of the age-adjusted range

**Why it matters:** DHEA-S is your adrenal androgen precursor. Low levels often correlate with the burnout pattern, chronic fatigue, low stress tolerance, and feeling like your battery never fully charges. In perimenopause and post-menopause, your adrenals become your primary hormone source, so DHEA-S reflects how well that backup system is functioning.

### Sex Hormone Binding Globulin (SHBG)

- Normal: 18 to 144 nmol/L
- Optimal: 60 to 80 nmol/L

**Why it matters:** SHBG binds sex hormones and controls how much is bioavailable. Low SHBG means more free testosterone circulating, which can show up as acne, hair loss, and insulin resistance. High SHBG means less bioavailable estrogen and testosterone, even if total levels look normal. This is the number that explains why your hormones look fine on paper but you still feel terrible.

### Cortisol (AM serum or 4-point salivary)

- Normal (AM serum): 6 to 23 µg/dL
- Optimal (AM serum): 10 to 18 µg/dL

**Why it matters:** Cortisol is your stress hormone, and it directly competes with progesterone for the same precursor, pregnenolone. Chronic cortisol elevation means less raw material for progesterone production, which is why high stress and terrible luteal phases go hand in hand. A 4-point salivary cortisol or DUTCH cortisol panel shows your daily rhythm, not just a single morning number. This is especially important in perimenopause when your adrenals are trying to compensate for declining ovarian function.

### Fasting Insulin

- Normal: 2–25 uIU/mL
- Optimal: Less than 5 uIU/mL

**Why it matters:** Most labs will not flag insulin until it is above twenty-five, by which point insulin resistance is well-established. Optimal fasting insulin is below five. Insulin resistance disrupts ovulation, increases androgen production, worsens PCOS symptoms, and accelerates during perimenopause and menopause as estrogen's insulin-sensitizing effect declines. This is the metabolic marker that catches the problem years before a diabetes diagnosis.

### Fasting Glucose

- Normal: 70 to 99 mg/dL
- Optimal: 75 to 85 mg/dL

**Why it matters:** A fasting glucose of ninety-eight is technically normal. It is also trending toward insulin resistance. Pair this with fasting insulin for the full metabolic picture. If glucose is creeping up while insulin is also elevated, your body is working harder to maintain blood sugar control.

### ▣ hs-CRP (High Sensitivity C-Reactive Protein)

- Normal: Less than 3.0 mg/L
- Optimal: Less than 1.0 mg/L

**Why it matters:** hs-CRP is a systemic inflammation marker and an independent cardiovascular risk factor. Rising inflammation during perimenopause and post-menopause drives joint pain, brain fog, mood instability, and cardiovascular risk. If your hs-CRP is climbing while your hormones are shifting, inflammation is compounding the problem.

### ▣ Homocysteine

- Normal: 5 to 15 umol/L
- Optimal: 6 to 9 umol/L

**Why it matters:** Elevated homocysteine signals sluggish methylation, the process that drives neurotransmitter production, estrogen detoxification, and DNA repair. Women with high homocysteine often struggle with anxiety, mood instability, and perimenopausal symptoms because their bodies cannot efficiently clear used hormones or produce new neurotransmitters.

### ▣ Magnesium (RBC)

- Normal: 4.2 to 6.8 mg/dL
- Optimal: 5.5 to 6.5 mg/dL

**Why it matters:** Serum magnesium is nearly useless because your body will pull magnesium from cells to keep serum levels stable. RBC magnesium reflects your true intracellular stores. Low magnesium contributes to anxiety, muscle cramps, insomnia, migraines, and poor stress tolerance. It is one of the most common deficiencies and one of the easiest to address.

### RBC Folate

- Normal: Greater than 200 ng/mL
- Optimal: Greater than 400 ng/mL

**Why it matters:** Folate keeps estrogen metabolism on track, supports methylation, and reduces PMS severity. Low folate impairs serotonin and dopamine production and worsens mood instability around ovulation and the luteal phase.

### AMH (Anti-Mullerian Hormone)

- Normal: 1.0 to 3.5 ng/mL during reproductive years (age- dependent, declines over time)

**Why it matters:** AMH tracks ovarian reserve. It is not diagnostic on its own, but it helps map where you are in the perimenopausal transition. Rapidly declining AMH alongside rising FSH paints a clear picture of accelerating ovarian aging.

### ▨ Estrone (E1)

- Normal (post-menopause): 10 to 60 pg/mL

**Why it matters:** Estrone becomes the dominant estrogen after menopause and is primarily produced in fat tissue. Elevated estrone with low estradiol may indicate poor estrogen metabolism. This ratio matters for both symptom management and long-term risk assessment.

### ▨ DUTCH Complete (Dried Urine Test for Comprehensive Hormones)

This is not a single marker but a comprehensive panel that measures hormone metabolites through dried urine collection over a twenty-four-hour period. It shows how your body produces, metabolizes, and clears estrogen, progesterone, testosterone, cortisol, and their downstream pathways. The estrogen metabolite breakdown (2-OH, 4-OH, 16-OH) is especially valuable during perimenopause because it reveals whether your body is clearing estrogen safely or routing it through pathways associated with increased risk. If you can access one test beyond standard serum labs, this is the one.

## ☑ Moving On

Now that you understand the hormonal operating system running beneath everything else in this book, there is one more piece to lock in before we move on. Your hormones set the rhythm, but your thyroid sets the speed. It controls how fast your brain fires, how efficiently you produce neurotransmitters, and how well every system we just talked about runs. In the next chapter, we are pulling back the curtain on the butterfly gland and the labs your doctor probably skipped.

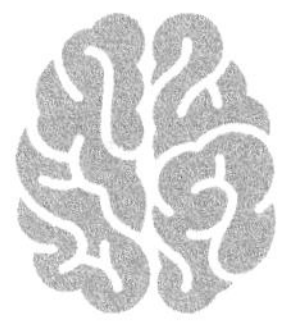



# CHAPTER 10

# THE BUTTERFLY GLAND WITH A GOD COMPLEX: YOUR THYROID AND YOUR BRAIN

If your hormones are the operating system, your thyroid is the processor. It sets the speed at which everything else runs. And when it slows down, it does not send you a notification.

## What Your Thyroid Actually Does

Your thyroid is a butterfly shaped gland that sits at the base of your throat, and it controls the metabolic rate of virtually every cell in your body. That includes your brain cells. It regulates how fast your neurons fire, how efficiently you produce neurotransmitters, how well you metabolize energy, how your body manages temperature, and how quickly you can think, process, and respond to the world around you.

When your thyroid is functioning well, you do not notice it. You have steady energy. Your mood is stable. Your hair grows. Your skin glows. Your digestion works. Your periods are regular. You can think clearly and remember what you walked into a room to get.

When your thyroid is struggling, everything dims. Not dramatically, not all at once, but slowly enough that you adjust. You start believing this is just how you are now. Tired. Foggy. Gaining weight for no reason. Losing hair in the shower. Constipated. Cold all the time. Depressed but not "depressed enough" for anyone to take seriously.

The most dangerous thing about thyroid dysfunction is not the symptoms. It is how slowly they arrive. You do not notice the lights dimming when they go down one percent at a time.

## The Thyroid-Brain Connection

Your brain is one of the most thyroid-dependent organs in your body. Thyroid hormones cross the blood brain barrier and directly influence neurotransmitter production and receptor sensitivity. When thyroid hormones are low, serotonin production slows. Dopamine signaling weakens. GABA activity drops. The result is depression, anxiety, brain fog, poor concentration, and emotional flatness that looks like a mood disorder but is actually an endocrine problem.

This is not a subtle connection. Research consistently shows that subclinical hypothyroidism, where TSH is elevated but still technically within the reference range, is associated with higher rates of depression, anxiety, and cognitive decline in women. The brain does not care whether your labs are "in range." It cares whether it is getting enough T3 to function.

Here is the part that gets missed most often. Your thyroid produces primarily T4, which is the storage form of thyroid hormone. T4 is inactive. It has to be converted into T3, the active form, before your cells can use it. That conversion happens in your liver, your gut, and your peripheral tissues, and it requires adequate levels of selenium, zinc, iron, and vitamin D. It is also suppressed by chronic stress, systemic inflammation, gut dysbiosis, and caloric restriction.

So you can have a thyroid that is technically producing enough T4, a TSH that looks fine, and still be functionally hypothyroid at the cellular level because your body is not converting T4 into T3 efficiently. This is the gap that standard testing misses, and it is the gap where millions of women live.

If you have been told your thyroid is normal but you still feel like you are wading through cement, the problem may not be what your thyroid is making. It may be what your body is doing with it.

## Hashimoto's: The Autoimmune Piece

Hashimoto's thyroiditis is the most common autoimmune condition in women, and it is the most common cause of hypothyroidism in the developed world. In Hashimoto's, your immune system produces antibodies that attack your thyroid tissue, gradually destroying its ability to produce hormones.

What makes Hashimoto's particularly insidious is the timeline. You can have elevated antibodies for years, sometimes a decade, before your TSH moves out of range. During that time, you are symptomatic. You have fatigue, brain fog, anxiety, hair loss, joint pain, and mood swings. But because your TSH is still "normal," nobody checks antibodies, and you are told there is nothing wrong.

Hashimoto's also does not present in a straight line. In the early stages, as the immune system attacks the thyroid, stored hormone gets dumped into the bloodstream in bursts. This creates periods of hyperthyroid symptoms, anxiety, racing heart, insomnia, irritability, followed by crashes into hypothyroid territory. Women in this phase often get diagnosed with an anxiety disorder or told they are having panic attacks. They are not. Their immune system is dismantling their thyroid in waves, and the hormonal surges and drops are producing psychiatric symptoms.

If your anxiety comes and goes in unpredictable waves, if you swing between wired and exhausted with no pattern, and if your mood does not match your circumstances, check TPO antibodies. Hashimoto's mimics psychiatric conditions better than almost anything else in medicine.

## Why Women Get Hit Harder

Women are five to eight times more likely to develop thyroid disease than men. The reasons are rooted in the immune system, hormonal fluctuations, and the specific vulnerabilities that come with female biology.

Estrogen modulates immune function, and every major hormonal shift in a woman's life, puberty, pregnancy, postpartum, perimenopause, and menopause, can trigger or worsen autoimmune thyroid disease. Postpartum thyroiditis affects up to 10% of women and is one of the most underdiagnosed causes of postpartum depression and anxiety. Perimenopause is another high-risk window. As estrogen becomes erratic, the immune system destabilizes, and Hashimoto's that was quietly simmering can flare.

Pregnancy itself dramatically increases thyroid hormone demand. Your thyroid output needs to increase by roughly 50% to support fetal brain development, especially in the first trimester before the baby's thyroid is functional. Women with borderline thyroid function or undiagnosed Hashimoto's may decompensate during pregnancy, developing overt hypothyroidism that affects both their mental health and fetal neurodevelopment.

The postpartum period is equally critical. The immune suppression that protects the pregnancy reverses, and the resulting immune rebound can trigger Hashimoto's flares or new onset thyroiditis. A woman who was fine before pregnancy can develop autoimmune thyroid disease in the months after delivery and be told she is just adjusting to motherhood.

## The Thyroid and Your Other Hormones

Your thyroid does not operate in isolation. It is deeply connected to your adrenal function, your sex hormones, your insulin signaling, and your gut health. When one system goes down, the others feel it.

### Thyroid and Cortisol

Chronic stress suppresses thyroid function through multiple pathways. Elevated cortisol inhibits TSH secretion, reduces T4 to T3 conversion, and increases reverse T3 production. Reverse T3 is a metabolically inactive form of thyroid hormone that blocks active T3 from reaching your cells. Your labs can look normal while your cells are functionally starved. This is why women under chronic stress develop thyroid symptoms even when their panels look clean. The cortisol is quietly sabotaging the conversion process.

### Thyroid and Estrogen

Estrogen increases thyroid binding globulin, the protein that carries thyroid hormones through your blood. When estrogen is high, more thyroid hormone gets bound up and less is free to enter cells. This is why some women feel hypothyroid during the luteal phase of their cycle when estrogen is relatively elevated, or why thyroid symptoms can worsen on estrogen-containing birth control or HRT. It is also why thyroid function should be re-evaluated whenever you make a change to your hormonal contraception or start hormone replacement therapy.

### Thyroid and Insulin

Thyroid hormones directly affect insulin sensitivity and glucose metabolism. Hypothyroidism, even subclinical, impairs your body's ability to use insulin efficiently, which means you are more prone to blood sugar swings, energy crashes, and weight gain concentrated around your midsection. The reverse is also true. Insulin resistance impairs thyroid function. High insulin levels suppress TSH and reduce thyroid hormone conversion. This creates a bidirectional cycle where thyroid problems and metabolic problems reinforce each other.

## Thyroid and the Gut

Roughly 20% of T4 to T3 conversion happens in the gut, which means your microbiome directly influences your thyroid hormone levels. Gut dysbiosis, intestinal permeability, and chronic inflammation all impair conversion. Additionally, Hashimoto's is strongly associated with celiac disease, and non-celiac gluten sensitivity is a documented trigger for thyroid antibody production in susceptible individuals. If your thyroid antibodies are elevated, your gut is part of the investigation.

## What Standard Testing Misses

The standard thyroid screening in most primary care offices is a TSH. That is it. One number. And if that number falls between 0.5 and 4.5 mIU/L, you are told your thyroid is fine.

Here is what a TSH alone does not tell you. It does not tell you how much free T4 your thyroid is producing. It does not tell you how much T3 your body is making from that T4. It does not tell you whether reverse T3 is blocking your cells from receiving the signal. It does not tell you whether your immune system is destroying your thyroid. And it does not tell you whether the thyroid hormone you are making is actually reaching your brain.

A complete thyroid evaluation requires TSH, free T4, free T3, reverse T3, TPO antibodies, and thyroglobulin antibodies. Anything less is a partial picture. And a partial picture is how millions of women end up on antidepressants for what is actually a thyroid problem.

If your doctor only checks TSH and tells you your thyroid is fine, they have not checked your thyroid. They have checked one marker. That is like checking the oil light on your dashboard and declaring the entire engine is running perfectly.

## Nutrients Your Thyroid Needs

Your thyroid cannot function without specific raw materials, and deficiency in any of them will slow the entire system down.

- **Selenium** is required for the enzyme that converts T4 to T3. Without adequate selenium, you can produce all the T4 in the world and still be functionally hypothyroid. Selenium also helps regulate the immune response in Hashimoto's and has been shown to reduce TPO antibodies in multiple studies. Brazil nuts are the most concentrated food source. Two to three per day provides approximately 200 mcg.
- **Zinc** supports TSH production, T4 to T3 conversion, and thyroid receptor sensitivity. Low zinc is common in women who are vegetarian, under chronic stress, or taking oral contraceptives. Oysters, pumpkin seeds, and red meat are the best dietary sources.

- **Iron** is essential for thyroid peroxidase, the enzyme your thyroid uses to produce T4 in the first place. Low ferritin directly impairs thyroid hormone synthesis. If your ferritin is below 50 ng/mL, your thyroid is not getting what it needs, even if your hemoglobin and CBC look normal.

- **Iodine** is the backbone of thyroid hormone. T4 contains four iodine atoms and T3 contains three. Most women in developed countries get adequate iodine through iodized salt and dairy, but women who eat low sodium diets, avoid dairy, or consume large amounts of goitrogenic foods without cooking them may be borderline insufficient. However, excess iodine is equally harmful and can trigger Hashimoto's flares. Do not mega-dose iodine supplements without testing first.

- **Vitamin D** modulates the immune system and is consistently low in women with Hashimoto's. Maintaining vitamin D between 50 and 70 ng/mL supports both thyroid function and immune regulation.

- **Magnesium** supports T4 to T3 conversion and is depleted by stress, caffeine, and sugar. Most women are deficient. RBC magnesium is the test that matters, not serum.

## What to Do With This Information

If you have been struggling with fatigue, brain fog, depression, anxiety, hair loss, weight gain, irregular cycles, or cold intolerance and your thyroid has only been evaluated with a TSH, you have not been fully evaluated. Request the complete panel. TSH, free T4, free T3, reverse T3, TPO antibodies, and thyroglobulin antibodies.

If your provider resists running the full panel, advocate for yourself. Bring this chapter. Explain why a single TSH is insufficient. If they still refuse, find a provider who will run it, or order the panel yourself through a direct-to-consumer lab service.

If your results come back and everything is "in range" but you still feel terrible, look at where your numbers fall within the range. A TSH of 3.8 is not the same as a TSH of 1.5, even though both are technically normal. A free T3 of 2.4 is not the same as a free T3 of 3.5. Optimal is not a range. It is a target, and your symptoms are the evidence of whether you are hitting it.

Your thyroid is the engine behind your energy, your mood, your cognition, and your capacity to show up for your life. Treat it accordingly.

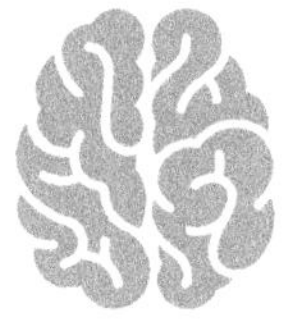



# TL;DR, DO THIS NOW, AND CLINICAL CUES

## ☑ TL;DR

Your thyroid controls the metabolic speed of every cell in your body, including your brain. When it slows down, serotonin drops, dopamine weakens, GABA falls, and you end up fatigued, foggy, anxious, depressed, and gaining weight while being told your labs are fine. The standard screening, a TSH alone, misses the full picture. You can have a normal TSH while your body fails to convert storage hormone (T4) into active hormone (T3), while reverse T3 blocks what little T3 you have, and while your immune system quietly destroys your thyroid tissue through Hashimoto's. Women are five to eight times more likely to develop thyroid disease, and every major hormonal transition, puberty, postpartum, perimenopause,

menopause, can trigger or worsen it. Chronic stress, gut dysfunction, and nutrient deficiencies all impair thyroid function even when the gland itself is intact.

## ☑ Do This Now

Request a complete thyroid panel at your next appointment. That means TSH, free T4, free T3, reverse T3, TPO antibodies, and thyroglobulin antibodies. Not just TSH. If your provider only wants to run TSH, advocate for the full panel or order it yourself through a direct-to-consumer service. While you are at it, check your ferritin, vitamin D, selenium (if available), and magnesium RBC, because your thyroid cannot function without these raw materials. If you are already on thyroid medication and still feel terrible, ask your provider to check free T3 and reverse T3 specifically. You may be making enough T4 but not converting it, and that distinction changes the treatment approach entirely.

## ☑ Clinical Cues

This guide helps you read your thyroid labs the way a clinician does. "Normal" is the broad reference interval printed on your lab report. "Optimal" is where most women feel and function their best. Use these cues to understand your own results and to catch the gap between "technically fine" and actually fine.

### ▧ TSH (Thyroid Stimulating Hormone)

- Normal: 0.4 to 4.5 mIU/L
- Optimal: 1.0 to 2.0 mIU/L

**Why it matters:** TSH is the signal your pituitary sends to your thyroid telling it to work. When TSH rises, it means the brain is yelling louder because the thyroid is not keeping up. A TSH of 3.8 is technically in range. It is not where your brain works well. Many women with TSH between 2.5 and 4.5 have textbook hypothyroid symptoms, fatigue, brain fog, weight gain, depression, and are told nothing is wrong. TSH alone also misses conversion problems, reverse T3 issues, and autoimmune thyroid disease. It is a starting point, not the full story.

### ▧ Free T4 (Thyroxine)

- Normal: 0.8 to 1.8 ng/dL
- Optimal: 1.0 to 1.5 ng/dL

**Why it matters:** Free T4 is the storage form of thyroid hormone, the raw material your body converts into active T3. Low free T4 with elevated TSH signals the thyroid gland itself is underproducing. But free T4 can also look normal while your body fails to convert it into usable T3, especially under chronic stress, inflammation, or nutrient deficiency. A normal free T4 without checking free T3 only tells you the factory has inventory. It does not tell you whether that inventory is reaching the cells that need it.

### Free T3 (Triiodothyronine)

- Normal: 2.3–4.2 pg/mL
- Optimal: 3.0 to 3.8 pg/mL

**Why it matters:** Free T3 is the active thyroid hormone. This is the one that actually enters your cells, drives energy production, regulates mood, and sharpens cognition. Low free T3 is one of the most common hidden drivers of treatment-resistant depression and chronic fatigue in women. Your TSH can be normal. Your T4 can be normal. And your free T3 can be sitting at 2.3, which means your cells are starved for the hormone that runs them. Chronic stress, gut inflammation, and deficiencies in selenium, zinc, and iron all impair the conversion of T4 into T3. If you have been told your thyroid is fine but you still feel like you are running on 30 percent battery, this is the number to fight for.

### Reverse T3 (rT3)

- Normal: 9.2 to 24.1 ng/dL
- Optimal: 9.2 to 14 ng/dL

**Why it matters:** Reverse T3 is your body's emergency brake. When you are chronically stressed, undereating, overtraining, inflamed, or running on cortisol fumes, your body converts T4 into rT3 instead of active T3. Reverse T3 is metabolically inactive and blocks active T3 from reaching your cells. Your TSH, T4, and even T3 can all look acceptable while rT3 quietly blocks the signal at the cellular level. The free T3 to reverse T3 ratio is what matters most. Divide your free T3 (in pg/mL) by your rT3 (in ng/dL). If the ratio is below 0.2, your cells are not getting thyroid hormone regardless of what your other numbers say. This is the test that catches women who are falling through the cracks of standard screening.

### ◾ TPO Antibodies (Thyroid Peroxidase Antibodies)

- Normal: Less than 35 IU/mL
- Optimal: Less than 10 IU/mL

**Why it matters:** Elevated TPO antibodies mean your immune system is attacking your thyroid tissue. This is Hashimoto's thyroiditis. You can have elevated antibodies for years before TSH ever moves out of range, which means you can be symptomatic, losing hair, exhausted, anxious, brain fogged, long before you meet the diagnostic criteria for hypothyroidism. Even "mildly" elevated antibodies above thirty-five signal ongoing immune-mediated inflammation that affects brain function, mood stability, and energy. If your mood swings do not match your hormone levels and your thyroid panel looks normal, this is the test being skipped. Perimenopause, postpartum, and any major hormonal transition are high-risk windows for Hashimoto's flares.

### Thyroglobulin Antibodies (TgAb)

- Normal: Less than 1 IU/mL (varies by lab, some use less than 4 IU/mL)

**Why it matters:** Thyroglobulin antibodies are the other half of the autoimmune thyroid picture. Some women with Hashimoto's have elevated TgAb but normal TPO, which means checking only TPO can miss the diagnosis. If you suspect autoimmune thyroid disease and your TPO comes back clean, request TgAb before ruling it out.

### Selenium (serum or whole blood)

- Normal: 70 to 150 ng/mL
- Optimal: 100 to 130 ng/mL

**Why it matters:** Selenium is required for the enzyme (deiodinase) that converts T4 into T3. Without adequate selenium, conversion slows and you become functionally hypothyroid even with normal TSH and T4. Selenium also modulates the immune response and has been shown to reduce TPO antibodies in women with Hashimoto's. Two to three Brazil nuts per day provides roughly 200 mcg, which is enough for most women. Do not exceed 400 mcg daily from all sources, as selenium toxicity is real.

### Zinc (serum or RBC)

- Normal: 60 to 120 μg/dL
- Optimal: 90 to 110 μg/dL

**Why it matters:** Zinc supports TSH production, T4 to T3 conversion, and thyroid receptor sensitivity. Low zinc impairs your thyroid at multiple levels. Women who are vegetarian, under chronic stress, or taking oral contraceptives are at higher risk for depletion. Zinc also competes with copper for absorption, so long-term supplementation should include periodic copper monitoring.

### Ferritin

- Normal: 12 to 150 ng/mL
- Optimal: 50 to 100 ng/mL

**Why it matters:** Iron is essential for thyroid peroxidase, the enzyme your thyroid needs to produce T4. Low ferritin directly impairs thyroid hormone synthesis, which means you can have a structurally healthy thyroid that simply cannot produce enough hormone because it does not have the iron to do so. A ferritin of eighteen is normal. It is also low enough to impair both thyroid function and energy production. This is one of the most common overlapping deficiencies in women with hypothyroid symptoms.

### ▨ Vitamin D (25-OH)

- Normal: 30 to 100 ng/mL
- Optimal: 50 to 70 ng/mL

**Why it matters:** Vitamin D is an immune modulator, and it is consistently low in women with Hashimoto's. Low vitamin D is associated with higher TPO antibody levels and more symptomatic thyroid disease. Maintaining optimal vitamin D supports immune regulation and may slow the autoimmune destruction of thyroid tissue.

### ▨ Cortisol (AM serum or 4-point salivary)

- Normal (AM serum): 6 to 23 µg/dL
- Optimal (AM serum): 10 to 18 µg/dL

**Why it matters:** Elevated cortisol suppresses TSH secretion, inhibits T4 to T3 conversion, and increases reverse T3 production. This is the direct mechanism by which chronic stress causes thyroid symptoms even when the thyroid gland itself is healthy. If your reverse T3 is elevated and your free T3 is low, cortisol is almost certainly part of the picture. A 4-point salivary cortisol or DUTCH cortisol panel will show you the full daily rhythm.

### ▪ Magnesium (RBC)

- Normal: 4.2 to 6.8 mg/dL
- Optimal: 5.5 to 6.5 mg/dL

**Why it matters:** Magnesium supports T4 to T3 conversion and is depleted by stress, caffeine, sugar, and hormonal fluctuations. Low magnesium compounds thyroid dysfunction by impairing conversion while also worsening anxiety, muscle cramps, and insomnia. Always test RBC magnesium, not serum.

## ☑ Moving On

You now understand the two systems running the show beneath everything else in this book: your reproductive hormones and your thyroid. They set the speed, the mood, and the capacity for everything that comes next. Before we move on, let's lock it in. The next section is a quick recap of everything you just learned about your cycle, your hormones, and the butterfly gland with a god complex. Think of it as the highlight reel before we keep building.

# PART 2 RECAP:
# KNOW YOUR OPERATING SYSTEM

Every hormone shift, every thyroid slowdown, every conversion problem you just learned about directly drains your nervous system's load capacity. When your progesterone tanks in the luteal phase, your GABA drops with it, and suddenly your stress tolerance disappears. When your thyroid is not converting T4 into T3, your brain is running on reduced power, burning through capacity just to maintain baseline function. When your estrogen becomes erratic in perimenopause, your serotonin and dopamine follow, and the mood instability is not a character flaw. It is a measurable biochemical event. This is why these chapters matter: every hormonal and thyroid deficit you identify and address restores capacity. You are not just learning biology.

You are reclaiming bandwidth. A quick review:

## Chapter 9: Your Cycle, Perimenopause, Menopause, and Your Brain

Your menstrual cycle is a monthly neurochemical reset. Estrogen and progesterone directly modulate serotonin, dopamine, and GABA, which means every phase of your cycle changes how your brain works.

Perimenopause can start in your mid-thirties and last a decade. Anxiety, brain fog, rage, insomnia, and weight gain are not stress. They are erratic hormone ratios your labs can quantify.

Menopause settles hormones at a permanently low baseline.

The first five years carry the steepest bone density decline and sharpest cardiovascular risk increase.

"Normal" labs do not mean optimal function. The gap between in range and feeling like yourself is where the real conversation starts.

## Chapter 10: The Butterfly Gland with a God Complex: Your Thyroid and Your Brain

Your thyroid sets the metabolic speed of every cell in your body, including your neurons. When it slows, serotonin drops, dopamine weakens, and cognition dims so gradually you think it is just who you are now.

A TSH alone is not a thyroid evaluation. You need TSH, free T4, free T3, reverse T3, TPO antibodies, and thyroglobulin antibodies for the full picture.

Hashimoto's can produce symptoms for years before TSH moves out of range. It mimics anxiety disorders, depression, and panic attacks. TPO antibodies are the test being skipped.

Chronic stress, gut dysfunction, and nutrient deficiencies (selenium, zinc, iron, vitamin D, magnesium) all impair thyroid function even when the gland itself is healthy.

## Integration Time and Moving On

You now have the full biochemical map. You understand what your body needs to eat, how your hormones shape your mood and cognition across every phase of life, and why your thyroid is the engine that determines whether any of it actually runs. You know which labs to request, what optimal looks like versus what "normal" hides, and why a single TSH or a single hormone draw is never the whole story.

The goal is not to fix everything at once. Start with the system screaming the loudest.

Maybe your luteal phase has been wrecking you for years and nobody has checked your progesterone on day twenty-one.

Maybe your TSH came back at 3.5 and you were told you were fine while your hair fell out in the shower.

Maybe your ferritin is 18 and the only reason you are still upright is caffeine and willpower.

Get the labs. Read the numbers. Track the trends. Use the Lab Tracker at the back of this book. Your body has been sending you data for years. Now you know how to read it.

# PART 3

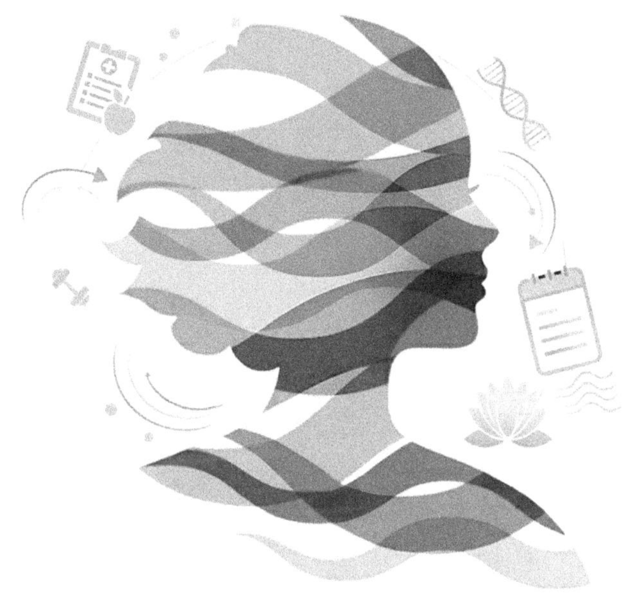

# MOVE YOUR MIND— THE SCIENCE AND SOUL OF SWEAT

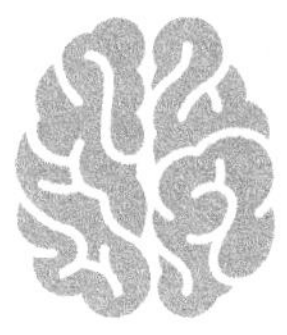



# CHAPTER 11

# WHY WE NEED TO MOVE (EVEN WHEN WE'RE TIRED, BUSY, OR JUST DON'T WANNA)

## The Evolution of Movement: Why Our Brains Are Built for Bodies in Motion

The evolutionary reality check: Our bodies were designed for movement—hunting, gathering, walking miles daily. Ergonomic desk chairs, midday scrolls, and three-tap Thai food delivery? That's new. For 99.9% of human history, "exercise" was just life. If you didn't move, you didn't eat. Or survive. Or avoid being eaten by something with more teeth than social tact.

Movement was the original multi-tool: It kept the body fueled, the brain alert, and the species alive. Our brains evolved to reward physical activity with feel-good chemicals because movement literally meant survival. You chased food, found water, gathered your tribe, and your brain said, "Good job! Here's a shot of dopamine."

Fast-forward to now, where the most physical effort required in a day might be fighting with a fitted sheet or opening a pickle jar. The reward system? Still hardwired to movement. But when you're not moving? No dopamine for you.

## Evolutionary Mismatch: The Caveman in a Cubicle

Imagine dropping a barefoot, spear-wielding hunter–gatherer into a modern office cubicle. She's suddenly surrounded by blue light, processed snacks, and ergonomic chairs. Her instincts are screaming, *"Move! Forage! Hunt! Run!"* But instead, she's told to sit, type, and check Slack. That mismatch goes deeper than physical discomfort; it's biological betrayal.

Our ancestors moved to survive. Now we survive by sitting still, clicking buttons, and outsourcing motion to machines. Our neurochemistry still expects constant movement. We're still wired to feel good *after* effort, not before.

When we stop moving, it's like asking Stone Age biology to handle Silicon Valley ergonomics. The system crashes slowly, and often silently through mental health symptoms, fatigue, and the gnawing sense that something's . . . off.

So if you've ever felt vaguely anxious after sitting still for seven hours straight, congratulations, you're biologically intact. Your brain is gently (or loudly) screaming, "We were not built for this!"

## Sedentary Stress: How Stillness Steals Our Joy

The sedentary lifestyle is the overpriced knockoff handbag of modern life. It looks convenient, but it's held together by denial and bad stitching. Sitting is the new smoking, except without the vintage glamor or rebellious aesthetic. Stillness threatens physical health and sabotages mental well-being.

When you're parked on the couch or slouched in a chair all day, your body's natural systems—circulation, digestion, lymphatic drainage, even brain function—start to power down like a 2006 MacBook. Blood flow slows. Cortisol (your stress hormone) sticks around like a toxic ex. And joy? Joy has left the chat.

## Your Brain Has a Plumbing System

Movement powers your brain's cleaning crew beyond the typical endorphin rush. The *glymphatic system* (your brain's version of the lymphatic system) clears out waste, toxins, and even early signs of neurodegeneration, *but only if you move your body*. So yes, a walk can literally help your brain detox.

Movement helps regulate emotions, dissipate stress hormones, and produce neurotransmitters that make you feel more human. Stillness, on the other hand, keeps your body trapped in a low-key physiological panic. You may not *feel* panicked, but your nervous system thinks you're frozen in the forest, waiting to be eaten. Again, evolution.

## Tiny Movements, Big Impact: The NEAT Effect

Not all movement has to be a "workout." In fact, the most underrated strategy for supporting mental health might be NEAT: non-exercise activity thermogenesis. It's the energy you burn (and the neurochemicals you activate) through everyday actions: fidgeting, pacing while on the phone, folding laundry, even taking the stairs.

NEAT keeps your blood moving, metabolism humming, and neurotransmitters flowing. Think of it as micromovement therapy. Skip the gym membership. Find reasons to stand up and move throughout your day.

---

### EXPERT NOTE

Research from Dr. Genevieve Healy's lab at University of Queensland shows that prolonged sedentary time is associated with a roughly 20% increased risk of depression.

---

## Case Study: From Couchbound Chaos to Nervous System Nirvana

**"I didn't know I was stressed . . . until I started moving again."**
Sophie, thirty-six, marketing director, perfectionist, and serial sitter

- *Symptoms:* Anxiety, irritability, brain fog, poor sleep, and the emotional resilience of a soggy tissue
- *Lifestyle:* More than ten hours per day at a desk, "relaxes" by scrolling and doom-watching true crime, swears she's too "mentally tired" to work out

### The Hidden Stress of Stillness

When Sophie came to me, she was convinced she had adrenal fatigue or some rare hormonal disorder because "I'm tired, wired, and weird all the time." She was evolutionarily mismatched.

Her cortisol rhythm was jacked (hello, 3 a.m. panic wakings), her heart rate variability was in the toilet, and she hadn't exercised in months. Her brain had adapted to sitting still . . . and panicking about it.

"I didn't feel stressed," she said. "But I also had a tension headache for three weeks straight, so . . . "

### The Prescription: Movement, but Make It Gentle

Instead of slapping her with a gym-bro boot camp, we started with small, attainable goals.

- Ten-minute morning walks (sunlight + motion = natural cortisol regulation)
- 1 p.m. movement snack (two to five minutes: stretching, squats, or walking a flight of stairs)
- Evening yin yoga twice a week (for GABA support and parasympathetic activation)
- Dance breaks when her brain felt like soup

No HIIT. No shame spirals. Just motion that felt doable.

## The Results (in Less Than Four Weeks)

- Sleep improved by end of week one
- Afternoon crashes disappeared
- Anxiety decreased without meds
- Bowel movements got regular (movement = motility, baby)
- She felt "happier for no reason" and started craving more movement

## What We Learned

- You don't have to be "fit" to feel better; you just have to move like your body was designed to.
- Even micromovements rewire your brain's threat response and reengage feel-good neurotransmitters.
- When Sophie stopped outsourcing *all* movement to machines, her nervous system exhaled.

## Nerd Note: The Science Behind It

Studies show that:

- Just ten minutes of moderate movement can increase dopamine and serotonin.
- Movement stimulates BDNF (brain-derived neurotrophic factor), a protein that improves brain plasticity, focus, and mood.
- Low heart rate variability (HRV), a sign of poor stress resilience, can improve with just three to four weeks of consistent low-intensity movement.
- One 2017 study [Rebar et al., *American Journal of Preventive Medicine*] found that depressive symptoms fell by 26% in less than a month among people who shifted from inactive to moderately active.

## The Mental Health Cost of Convenience Culture

Convenience culture has taught us that faster is better, effort is optional, and anything that requires a smidge of sweat is either outdated or barbaric. Why walk when you can have a burrito drone-delivered to your door while you lie motionless in athleisure you haven't moved in since Monday?

Push-button luxury outpaced our evolutionary biology. Our bodies are still expecting us to do things: to lift, squat, reach, stretch, walk, climb, stir, carry, and when we don't, they revolt. Slowly. Silently. Psychologically.

Depression, anxiety, brain fog, poor sleep, irritability: these often reflect your nervous system's asking when you last saw the sun or moved your glutes.

Convenience is killing our mood because it eliminates the friction that used to keep us healthy. Making food, walking to a friend's house, even cleaning, all were built-in micromovements that served as physical maintenance. Now we have convenience without consequence until, of course, the consequence manifests as mental stagnation, emotional numbness, or the urge to scream into a pillow because your Amazon package is late.

Bottom line: We need to move. And getting started can be much, much easier than you think.

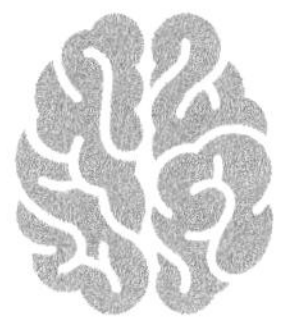



# TL;DR, DO THIS NOW, AND CLINICAL CUES

## ☑ TL;DR

- Our bodies evolved to move, not sit.
- Stillness disrupts hormone balance, neurotransmitter function, and emotional regulation.
- Movement (even light!) = more dopamine, less stress, better sleep.
- Micromovements count. NEAT is your new best friend.

## ☑ Do This Now

- Take a ten-minute walk first thing tomorrow morning.
- Add a two- to five-minute "movement snack" to your afternoon.

- Turn music on and dance in your kitchen (science says it counts).
- No perfection. Just progress.

## ☑ Clinical Cues

### ▓ Fasting Glucose and Insulin

- Normal: glucose 70–99 mg/dL, insulin 2–25 µIU/mL
- Optimal: glucose 75–85 mg/dL, insulin <5 µIU/mL

**Why it matters:** Movement improves insulin sensitivity. When these markers creep up, women often report fatigue, mood crashes, stubborn weight, and PMS that feels worse month by month. Even light movement stabilizes blood sugar and brain energy.

### ▓ HbA1c (three-month glucose average)

- Normal: <5.7%
- Optimal: 4.8–5.2%

**Why it matters:** Elevated A1c reflects chronically unstable blood sugar, which drives irritability, anxiety, and perimenopausal brain fog. Movement is one of the most powerful natural A1c regulators.

## High-Sensitivity C-Reactive Protein (hs-CRP)

- Normal: <3 mg/L
- Optimal: <1 mg/L

**Why it matters:** Sedentary lifestyles raise inflammation; consistent movement lowers it. High CRP is often the hidden reason women feel "old and achy" before fifty.

## Cortisol (a.m./p.m.)

- Normal a.m. (8 a.m.): 6–23 µg/dL
- Normal p.m. (4–6 p.m.): 3–10 µg/dL
- Optimal rhythm: strong a.m. rise $\rightarrow$ gentle p.m. decline

**Why it matters:** Movement retrains this rhythm. Without it, cortisol becomes erratic-wired at night, tanked in the morning. Exercise helps smooth the curve, reducing anxiety, sleep disruption, and stress sensitivity.

## Brain-Derived Neurotrophic Factor (BDNF)

- A protein your brain produces to grow new neurons and strengthen existing connections, (research/lifestyle marker rather than routine lab).

**Why it matters:** Movement spikes BDNF, which acts like Miracle-Gro for neurons. Low BDNF is tied to depression, poor memory, and perimenopausal cognitive decline. Even a brisk walk can flip the switch.

## ☑ Moving On

So now you know why your body throws a tantrum when you sit too long and why even a five-minute walk can flip your mood switch. Movement isn't just about burning calories or chasing some "fit" ideal; it's your nervous system's way of hitting refresh, and the real magic happens inside your skull.

Every squat, stretch, or shimmy kicks off a neurochemical rave in your brain, one that makes you calmer, clearer, and just a little more human. Which brings us to the fun part: the behind-the-scenes mixologists—endorphins, dopamine, serotonin, and friends—shaking up the ultimate cocktail of calm. Let's pull back the curtain on your brain's favorite happy hour lineup.

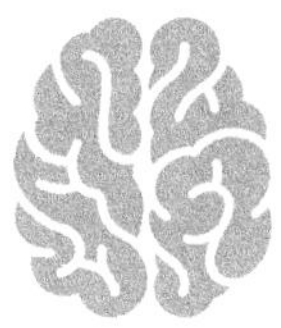



# ENDORPHINS, DOPAMINE, AND THE COCKTAIL OF CALM

Forget the vitamins you bought three months ago and never opened, and the therapy apps you're still auto-paying for because you forgot to cancel after the free trial. If you're reading this book, you're the kind of woman who wants to understand your brain chemistry and then actually do something with that knowledge. Good news: Your brain already comes stocked with a pharmacy. Today's special? Endorphins, dopamine, and the delightfully underrated neurochemical cocktail known as calm.

These molecules are the behind-the-scenes mixologists of your emotions, behaviors, and drive. Think of them as your inner bartenders: precise, moody, but surprisingly responsive to how you live your day.

## Endorphins: Nature's Tiny Painkillers with a Flair for Theatrics

Endorphins are neuropeptides released during stress or discomfort. They reduce pain and boost mood by binding to the brain's opioid receptors (but in a safe, nondestructive way).

Exercise? Triggers endorphins.

Laughter? Also endorphins.

Spicy food? You better believe it.

Even *anticipating* something exciting can spark a hit. [Stefano et al. (2005)] Evolution built them in to keep us going when survival required grit.

---

### EXPERT SIDEBAR:

"Endorphins are your brain's emergency chocolate stash; they show up when life gets tough and give you a boost you didn't know you needed."

---

## The Runner's High . . . Debunked (Sort Of)

We've been told endorphins are the reason for the runner's high. Reality check: Endorphins are too large to cross the blood–brain barrier. [Boecker et al. (2008)] If they can't enter the brain, they can't be responsible for that mood shift or post-run glow. The real secret weapon is endocannabinoids, your body's self-produced bliss molecules that work like cannabis without the THC. They do cross into the brain, binding to receptors that spark pleasure, calm, and flow. [Raichlen DA, Foster AD, Gerdeman GL, Seillier A, Giuffrida A." *Journal of Experimental Biology. 2012*] Translation? After a workout, your brain is essentially getting a mild, legal high.

And if you've never felt that high? That's completely normal. Some people feel euphoria; others experience subtle calm or mental clarity. The response varies, but your endocannabinoid system is still working.

## Dopamine: The Anticipation Architect

Dopamine works as your anticipation engine; the reward comes from expecting, not receiving. It spikes not when you *get* the reward, but when you *expect* it. [Volkow et al. (2011) *Molecular Psychiatry*] That's why checking your phone feels good even when it's just spam.

In a balanced brain, dopamine fuels motivation, progress, and joy in the *process*. In an imbalanced brain? It fuels obsession, distraction, and eventual exhaustion. Sound familiar?

Mini mental hack:

Dopamine thrives on *momentum,* so . . .

- Break goals into microsteps.
- Celebrate the tiny wins.
- Reduce digital dopamine junk food (scrolling, constant notifications).

If you reset your dopamine habits this way, every time you complete even a tiny action, like checking off "Drink water," your brain gives you a mini dopamine surge, its version of a standing ovation for follow-through.

## What Really Happens in Your Brain When You Exercise

Grab your highlighter; here's your biochemical cocktail menu:

Endorphins reduce physical discomfort. Dopamine gets you excited to move and rewards consistency. Endocannabinoids create that blissful calm. Serotonin regulates mood and energy. GABA quiets anxious overthinking post-workout.

This is simple science: Movement rewires your brain to be calmer, sharper, and more resilient.

---

**EXPERT SIDEBAR:**

"Exercise doesn't just change your body; it upgrades your brain. It mimics the effects of antidepressants by increasing serotonin and BDNF, often with fewer side effects."

---

## Movement Mimics Meds

Studies show aerobic exercise can be as effective as antidepressants in mild to moderate depression. [Blumenthal et al. (2007)] But consistency is the secret sauce. Five squats one time does not cancel therapy.

The inspiring part? Just twenty to thirty minutes of moderate activity most days creates measurable chemical shifts. And it doesn't have to be fancy:

- Walk your dog.
- Dance in your kitchen.
- Do yoga in pajama pants.

Your brain cares that you move, not how it looks.

## The Stress–Recovery Loop: How Your Brain Gets Better at Being Human

Your brain gets sharper, calmer, and more resilient through challenge and recovery. It adapts. It remodels. It upgrades itself based on the pressures you put it under, and the resources you give it to recover afterward. That cycle is called the stress–recovery loop, and it runs underneath everything in this book: movement, sleep, nutrients, hormones, inflammation, even how you think. The whole system, boiled down:

1. **Stressor:**

   A challenge asks your brain and body to perform. This could be a workout, a fasted morning walk, a heavy deadline, a new skill, a difficult emotional moment, or any stimulus that forces your system out of autopilot.

2. **Demand and Signal:**
Your nervous system reads the stressor as a call to upgrade. This is where BDNF rises, mitochondria multiply, neurotransmitter pathways recalibrate, and synapses get pruned or strengthened. The signal says, "Improve capacity so next time this isn't threatening."

3. **Repletion and Input:**
Recovery means rest plus raw materials. It's nutrients for neurotransmitter production, omega-3s for membranes, magnesium for calming circuits, sleep for consolidation, glucose stability for signal fidelity, and adequate protein so cellular remodeling can actually happen.

4. **Adaptation:**
If the system has enough raw materials, it responds:
   - HRV increases.
   - Mood stabilizes.
   - Cognitive flexibility improves.
   - Stress tolerance rises.
   - Inflammation drops.
   - Metabolic efficiency sharpens.

This is resilience, and it is earned biologically, not willed into existence.

**When the loop is broken:**

If you train, push, think, grind, and survive but never replenish, your body interprets every demand as a threat instead of an opportunity. Mood destabilizes. Recovery stalls. Anxiety spikes. Focus narrows into survival scanning. Your brain can only remodel upward when the stress is paired with fuel, rest, micronutrients, and metabolic stability.

**When the loop is intact:**

Movement becomes neuroplastic fertilizer, nutrition becomes structural material, sleep becomes code-writing time, and mindfulness becomes the steering wheel.

Stress becomes growth when your brain has the resources to adapt.

Everything in the chapters that follow—clinical labs, omega-3s, B vitamins, sleep phases, insulin curves—is part of that loop. They're the ingredients of your brain's adaptive machinery.

If you remember nothing else, remember this:

**Your brain doesn't thrive because life is easy. It thrives when challenge is paired with recovery.**

## The Cocktail of Calm: Serotonin, Oxytocin, and GABA

**Serotonin: The Mood Manager**

- Synthesized from tryptophan, serotonin regulates mood, sleep, appetite, and digestion. [Young (2007)] Balanced levels bring steadiness and clarity.

- Boost it with sunlight, tryptophan-rich foods (tofu, turkey, eggs), or mindfulness.

## Oxytocin: The Bond Builder

- Released during hugs, laughter, eye contact, and intimacy. It says, "We're better together."
- Boost it by cuddling, petting your pet, or looking someone in the eye instead of your phone.

## GABA: Your Brain's Chill Pill

- This neurotransmitter inhibits overactive neurons. It's the nervous system's equivalent of chamomile tea and weighted blankets.
- Boost it with deep breathing, slow yoga, or green tea's L-theanine.

## Cocktail Recipes for Your Nervous System

Here's how to mix and match your molecules without a lab coat:

- The Endorphin Shot: ten push-ups + hot sauce + belly laugh with a friend
- The Dopamine Spritz: check off a microtask + play your hype song
- The Calm-tini: five minutes of breath work + green tea + cuddle your dog

Your nervous system isn't picky; it just wants the ingredients.

> ## Case Study: Rewriting the Recipe
>
> "Maria," forty-two, attorney and single mom, told me she felt "chemically flat." She'd quit exercising, was running on caffeine, and said, "I can't remember the last time I felt joy.
>
> Instead of chasing a miracle pill, we rebuilt her cocktail:
>
> - Fifteen-minute morning walk (dopamine + serotonin)
> - Evening dance breaks with her kids (endorphins + oxytocin)
> - Nightly green tea ritual (GABA)
>
> In six weeks? Better sleep, fewer anxiety spikes, and spontaneous laughter she didn't have to force. Her words: "It feels like someone turned the lights back on in my brain."

## Final Thought

Skip the biohacking, expensive supplements, and marathon training. Your brain already holds the ingredients for calm, focus, and resilience; it just needs you to stir the shaker. You don't have to biohack, buy supplements, or go full marathoner. You simply have to mix your molecules with intention.

The lab is your life. The test subject is you. And this experiment? It's one you can actually win.

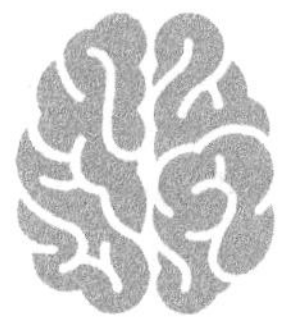



# TL;DR, DO THIS NOW, AND CLINICAL CUES

## ☑ TL;DR

- Endorphins ease discomfort, but endocannabinoids are the true stars behind the "runner's high." They switch on when you get your heart rate up for a bit (think brisk walking, jogging, or cycling).
- Dopamine thrives on momentum, so celebrate the tiny wins, not just the big ones.
- Exercise sparks a neurochemical cocktail: serotonin, GABA, dopamine, BDNF, and more.
- Oxytocin and GABA add connection and calm to the mix, and you don't need a gym membership to access them.
- Movement doesn't just change your body; it rewires your brain.

## ☑ Do This Now

- Pick one cocktail recipe for today:
    - Endorphin Shot (spicy food + quick movement + laughter)
    - Dopamine Spritz (tiny goal + hype song)
    - Calm-tini (breathwork + tea + hug your pet)
- Bonus: Write down one microgoal and check it off before the day ends. Your brain will thank you for the dopamine.

## ☑ Clinical Cues

### Fasting Glucose and Insulin

- Normal: glucose 70–99 mg/dL, insulin 2–25 µIU/mL
- Optimal: glucose 75–85 mg/dL, insulin <5 µIU/mL

**Why it matters:** Movement stabilizes glucose delivery to the brain. When insulin creeps up, dopamine signaling tanks → motivation and focus drop, PMS rage hits harder, and cravings spiral.

### HbA1c

- Normal: <5.7%
- Optimal: 4.8–5.2%

**Why it matters:** Long-term glucose balance = long-term neurotransmitter stability. Women with higher A1c often report irritability, anxiety, and "sluggish" thinking. Movement is medicine here.

### ▪ Organic Acids Test (OAT, functional lab)

- Markers: HVA (dopamine metabolite), 5-HIAA (serotonin metabolite), kynurenate/quinolinate (neuroinflammation markers)

**Why it matters:** Shows how well your body is actually producing and metabolizing neurotransmitters. Common in women: low dopamine turnover (no drive), high quinolinate (anxious/irritable), or low serotonin metabolites (PMS, insomnia). Movement shifts these patterns.

### ▪ Plasma Amino Acids (functional lab)

**Why it matters:** Tyrosine (dopamine precursor) and tryptophan (serotonin precursor) availability dictate how much raw material your brain has for mood chemistry. Functional medicine uses these to personalize nutrition + movement prescriptions.

### ▪ Cortisol and DHEA (four-point diurnal panel)

**Why it matters:** Exercise smooths cortisol spikes and raises DHEA, boosting resilience. Women with blunted cortisol curves, meaning their stress rhythm has lost its normal rise and fall, often feel unmotivated, depressed, or anxious until movement helps reset it.

## ☑ Moving On

You've got the ingredients lined up—endorphins, dopamine, serotonin, oxytocin, GABA—and you've even tried a cocktail or two. But here's the next step: learning how to shake, stir, and serve them in ways that specifically tackle stress, sharpen focus, and unlock that elusive flow state. Chapter 11 is where we stop winging it and start designing movement like it's personalized brain medicine. Because the truth is, not all movement hits your nervous system the same way, and knowing the difference is what turns "just exercise" into real emotional resilience.

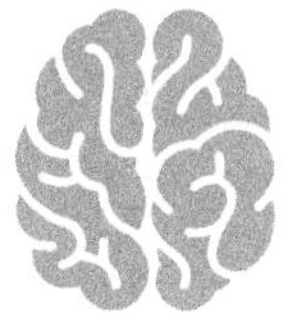



# IT'S NOT ABOUT THE GYM: REWRITING THE TOXIC FITNESS NARRATIVE

Thanks to social media and its algorithm-approved cult of grind culture, "working out" has been rebranded as punishment for existing in a human body. The phrase conjures images of grueling routines, sweat-drenched selfies, and a relentless pursuit of physical perfection.

What if movement became a celebration, not a chore? What if you stopped moving for a mirror and started moving for your nervous system?

## Movement Versus "Working Out"

Language shapes perception. When you shift from "working out" to "moving," you release yourself from obligation and open the door to joy.

Movement is about:

- Feeling good in your skin
- Regulating stress
- Building resilience
- Reminding your body you're alive and thriving

## Fun > Force: The Pleasure Principle of Movement

You're more likely to stick with habits that feel good. Choosing joy releases neurotransmitters like dopamine and endorphins, which elevate mood and reduce stress.

Dance, swim, walk, stretch, do tai chi; it all counts. And it all works better when you actually enjoy it.

The research backs this up:

- **Tai chi:** Improves depression, anxiety, and overall quality of life. [Huston and McFarlane (2016) *Canadian Family Physician*]
- **Yoga:** Consistently reduces symptoms of anxiety and depression, enhancing psychological well-being.
- **Micromovements:** Even five minutes of low-intensity activity can reduce cortisol and improve mood. [Reed and Ones (2019) Frontiers in Psychology]

## Case Study: Keisha's Ten-Minute Reset

Keisha, a thirty-eight-year-old middle school teacher and single mom, wasn't looking for transcendence. She just wanted ten minutes of not being needed.

One night, she rolled out a beach towel, bent forward, and breathed. Hamstrings screamed, leggings ripped, cat judged—but she kept showing up.

Within a week:

- She was snapping less at her kids.
- Her body didn't feel like a slinky.
- She stopped waking up clenched.

No job change. No guru. Just movement. Imperfect and consistent. And it rewired her nervous system from chaos to calm.

**Takeaway: Your body, a little space, and the radical belief you're worth ten minutes of care, that's all you need.**

## The Five-Minute Movement Prescription

If you've got five minutes, you've got medicine: short timed movements that reboot cortisol rhythm, lower muscle tension, and remind your nervous system you're safe.

## Quick Body Scan (thirty seconds)

- **What to do:** Sit tall. Scan from jaw to toes. Soften anything clenching.
- **Why it works:** This interrupts unconscious bracing patterns and drops muscle guarding that tells your brain "We're in danger." Releasing tension sends the opposite signal: "You're safe."

## Stretch and Sigh (one minute)

- **What to do:** Reach overhead, open the ribs, and exhale with a long audible sigh.
- **Why it works:** Expansion and slow exhale lengthens the diaphragm and taps the vagus nerve, lowering cortisol and shifting you toward rest-and-digest tone. You'll feel your shoulders drop, literally and neurologically.

## Wiggle It Out (one minute)

- **What to do:** Shake limbs lightly, sway, roll wrists, loosen jaw.
- **Why it works:** Shaking disperses built-up adrenaline, boosts circulation, and helps the motor cortex "reset" after hours of stillness. It's goofy on purpose: Breaking stiffness breaks threat perception.

## Cat-Cow (one minute)

- **What to do:** Round and arch the spine slowly while breathing deeply.

- **Why it works:** Mobilizing the spine lubricates spinal joints, opens rib movement, and stimulates spinal fluid flow. It wakes up the parts of your nervous system that stagnate when you sit.

**Breath Reset (one minute)**

- **What to do:** Inhale four counts, hold for four, exhale for six.
- **Why it works:** Lengthened exhale drives parasympathetic dominance, lowers heart rate, and tells the amygdala "No threat here." It's a mechanical off switch for stress chemistry. Your brain responds to micromessages of safety, not sweat equity.

## Weaving Movement into Real Life

The five-minute prescription works when you need structure. But movement doesn't have to live on a timer. Here's how to weave it into the moments you're already living:

- **At home:** Hip circles while your coffee brews, neck rolls during commercials, cat-cow before bed, chest opener when you wake up
- **At work:** Seated twist at your desk, wrist rolls between emails, forward fold during lunch, breathwork before meetings
- **In traffic (parked, not steering!):** Neck rolls, shoulder squeezes, box breathing

These are doorways, small moments where your body gets regular signals of activation without adding more to your plate.

## Bottom Line

Move on purpose. That's it. No CrossFit required.

Whether it's tai chi, chair stretches, or dancing in fuzzy socks, movement rewires your nervous system, boosts mood, and whispers to your body "Hey. You're safe. You're strong. You're still here."

The next time your brain doubts five minutes matters, remember this: Your nervous system measures signals, not duration. And five minutes of safety, release, and breath? That's a signal your body will absolutely receive.

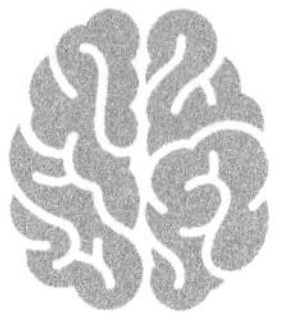

# CHAPTER 13.5

# TL;DR, DO THIS NOW, AND CLINICAL CUES

## ☑ TL;DR

- Movement ≠ punishment. Ditch "working out." Embrace *moving*.
- Consistency is built on rituals that feel good, not shame, not grind culture.
- Even five minutes of gentle movement can reset your nervous system.
- Keisha's story proves it: Ten minutes on a beach towel can transform a whole mood cycle.
- Your brain is dopamine driven: Habits that feel rewarding stick. Habits that feel like punishment don't.
- Every stretch, wiggle, or walk is a vote for your future self.

## ☑ Do This Now

Pick one of these micromovements today:

- The Stretch and Sigh (one minute): Arms up, lean, sigh dramatically. Nervous system gold.
- The Wiggle Reset (one minute): Shake arms, bounce heels, release static stress.
- Desk Twist (thirty seconds each side): Sneaky spinal reset mid-Zoom.
- Gratitude Reach (one minute): Reach arms overhead, breathe deeply, say something kind to yourself.

Bonus habit hack: Write down one movement you enjoyed today. Logging pleasure trains your brain to chase more of it.

## ☑ Clinical Cues

### ▦ Cortisol (four-point diurnal, saliva/urine)

- Normal a.m.: 6–23 µg/dL with steady decline to night
- Optimal: Strong a.m. rise with smooth taper by evening

**Why it matters:** Toxic "no days off" fitness spikes cortisol and keeps it high all day → anxiety, insomnia, cycle disruption. On the flip side, being sedentary flattens the curve. Balanced, Pleasure-based movement restores a healthy rhythm.

### ▪ DHEA-S

- Age-specific, optimal = upper half of reference range for age

**Why it matters:** Low in women who overtrain or are chronically stressed, leading to burnout, low libido, and depressed mood. Healthy, balanced exercise nudges DHEA up, restoring resilience.

### ▪ Creatine Kinase (CK, serum)

- Normal: 30–200 U/L (varies by lab)

**Why it matters:** Elevated CK can indicate muscle breakdown from overtraining. Women stuck in toxic workout cycles often live with chronically sore muscles, fatigue, and poor recovery masked as "discipline."

### ▪ Ferritin (iron storage)

- Normal: 12–150 ng/mL (women)
- Optimal: 50–100 ng/mL

**Why it matters:** Heavy training + poor recovery drains iron. Low ferritin = fatigue, irritability, hair loss. Women often push harder at the gym when they really need iron repletion and rest.

### Thyroid Panel

○ **TSH:**

- Normal: 0.4–4.0 mIU/L
- Optimal: 1.0–2.0 mIU/L

**Why it matters:** TSH is the screening test. A TSH of 3.5 is technically fine on paper, but many women at that level report fatigue, weight gain, brain fog, and depression that nobody can explain. Your pituitary sends TSH to tell your thyroid to work harder. When TSH creeps above 2.0, your thyroid is already struggling to keep up. Women in their thirties to fifties often get told "your thyroid is fine" while sitting at 3.0+ with textbook hypothyroid symptoms. A single TSH also misses the full picture, which is why free T3 and T4 matter too.

○ **Free T4:**

- Normal: 0.8–1.8 ng/dL
- Optimal: 1.0–1.5 ng/dL

**Why it matters:** T4 is the storage form of thyroid hormone, the raw material your body converts into active T3. Low free T4 means the factory is underproducing. You'll feel it as sluggish metabolism, depressed mood, dry skin, and the kind of fatigue that sleep doesn't fix. T4 can look "normal" while your body quietly fails to convert it into usable T3, especially under chronic stress, inflammation, or low selenium and zinc.

- **Free T3:**

  - Normal: 2.3–4.2 pg/mL
  - Optimal: 3.0–3.8 pg/mL

**Why it matters:** This is the hormone that actually does the work. T3 drives energy production, mood regulation, and cognitive sharpness at the cellular level. Low free T3 is one of the most common hidden drivers of treatment-resistant depression and chronic fatigue in women. Your TSH and T4 can both look fine while T3 sits low, meaning your cells are starving for fuel your labs say you have. Stress, gut inflammation, and nutrient deficiencies (especially selenium and zinc) all impair the T4-to-T3 conversion. If you've been told "your thyroid is normal" but you still feel like you're wading through cement, this is the marker to fight for.

- **Reverse T3 (rT3)**

  - Normal: 9.2–24.1 ng/dL
  - Optimal: 9.2–14 ng/dL

**Why it matters:** Reverse T3 is your body's emergency brake on metabolism. When you're chronically stressed, undereating, overtraining, inflamed, or running on cortisol fumes, your body converts T4 into rT3 instead of active T3. It's the biological equivalent of your nervous system saying, "We're in survival mode, shut it down." Your TSH, T4, and even T3 can all look acceptable while rT3 quietly blocks thyroid hormone from reaching your cells. Women who feel hypothyroid with "normal" labs often have elevated rT3. The free T3-to-reverse T3 ratio is what functional clinicians actually look at. If your ratio is below 0.2 (free T3 in pg/mL divided by rT3 in ng/dL), your cells aren't getting the thyroid signal no matter what the other numbers say. This is the lab that catches the women falling through the cracks.

## TPO Antibodies:

- Normal: <35 IU/mL
- Optimal: <10 IU/mL

**Why it matters:** Elevated TPO means your immune system is attacking your own thyroid. This is Hashimoto's thyroiditis, the most common autoimmune condition in women, and it can drive mood instability, anxiety, and depression long before TSH ever moves out of range. Even "mildly" elevated antibodies signal ongoing inflammation that affects brain function. Women often cycle between hypo and hyper symptoms for years before anyone thinks to check TPO. If your mood swings don't match your hormones and your thyroid labs look "fine," this is the test being skipped.

## ☑ **Moving On**

You've redefined movement as medicine, not punishment. You've learned that five minutes of dancing in your kitchen counts just as much as an hour at the gym and maybe even more, because it actually sticks. But here's the next layer: While solo movement heals, shared movement multiplies the magic. When we move with others, our bodies don't just get stronger; our nervous systems sync, our brains release bonding chemicals, and we remember that we were never meant to do this alone.

Which brings us to the underestimated secret weapon for mental health: community, connection, and the psychology of shared sweat.

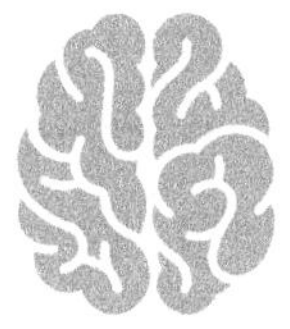



# CHAPTER 14

# COMMUNITY, CONNECTION, AND THE PSYCHOLOGY OF SHARED SWEAT

Welcome to one of the most underrated mental health interventions of all time: moving with other humans. Group exercise is therapy in motion except with better playlists, brighter leggings, and zero co-pays.

Sure, solo workouts have their place (no one needs to witness you accidentally uppercutting yourself during a YouTube kickboxing class). But there's something biologically and emotionally healing about moving in sync with other people. This is neuroscience, not just camaraderie.

## Group Movement as Mental Medicine

When you step into a spin class, a yoga studio, or even a neighborhood walking group, your brain is doing more than keeping pace. It's engaging in co-regulation, the syncing of nervous systems in shared environments. Think of it as emotional Bluetooth.

Moving with others floods your brain with dopamine (motivation), endorphins (pain relief and euphoria), and oxytocin (social bonding). Add in a fist bump or a post-Zumba hug, and your brain gets a reminder: "I belong here."

A 2017 study in the American Osteopathic Association's *Journal of Osteopathic Medicine* proves it. The study found that people in group exercise reported a 26% reduction in perceived stress, compared to just 11% in solo exercisers.

And in 2023, the US Surgeon General declared loneliness a public health epidemic, comparing its risks to smoking fifteen cigarettes a day. Group movement is medicine for a disconnected world.

Every time you high-five a workout buddy, hug a yoga friend, or fist-bump your trainer, you get a hit of oxytocin, the trust hormone. Small, safe touches lower stress and reinforce belonging. Your nervous system responds to small gestures. A handshake works. So does a sweaty side hug.

**EXPERT SIDEBAR:**

"Group exercise isn't just about fitness. It satisfies our primal need to connect through rhythm and shared effort. Humans are social creatures, and when we move together, we reinforce that bond physiologically and emotionally."

## Mirror Neurons and Motivation by Osmosis

Ever notice how watching someone in your class go all-in suddenly makes you push harder? That's mirror neurons at work. These brain cells fire when you act and when you watch someone else act. They're why yawns are contagious, why you flinch when someone ducks, and why burpees suck slightly less when the whole room is doing them too.

Shared effort creates shared energy. Music, rhythm, and breath amplify it. That collective "we're in this together" buzz lives in your neurons, literally.

## The Secret Intimacy of Walking-and-Talking

Not into group classes? Walking with a friend might be one of the most therapeutic forms of movement you'll ever try.

Walking side by side (instead of sitting across from each other with forced eye contact) creates a softer, more open channel for sharing. The rhythm regulates your breath and nervous system, while the forward motion sends your brain the message "We're moving through this together."

Therapists now use "walk-and-talk" sessions for this exact reason. Motion unlocks emotion.

## Practical Ways to Add Shared Movement

If you're already maxed out on time and energy, here's the low-lift menu:

- Join a virtual class with friends, and keep the cameras off. No makeup, no pressure.
- Walk with a coworker on lunch break and call it a "moving meeting."
- Start a group chat called Stretch Club and send proof-of-life photos of your toes.
- Do "errand walks" with a friend. Bank, pharmacy, gossip, done.
- Not a gym person? Try hiking clubs, dance nights, faith-based walking groups, even concerts where you just let your body move to music.

Community movement just has to be shared. Fancy? Optional.

## Hormones, Women, and the Moving Body

Behind the burpees and barre moves, another rhythm is happening inside you: your hormones. Estrogen, progesterone, cortisol, all of them influence how you feel, how you sleep, and how you show up to movement.

For women over thirty, exercise manages hormonal shifts with a little sweat and a lot of grace. Exercise regulates cortisol, boosts serotonin, and balances insulin sensitivity. It even helps smooth out PMS symptoms like cramps, mood swings, and fatigue.

The key? Working with your body's natural rhythms instead of against them.

## Working With Your Cycle Instead of Against It

- **Follicular phase (days one to fourteen-ish):** Rising estrogen means rising energy. Great for HIIT, spin, and strength training.
- **Ovulation:** Peak power. You'll feel strong and social. Hello, dance class.
- **Luteal phase (pre-period):** Progesterone climbs, energy dips. Switch to walking, yoga, or Pilates.
- **Menstruation:** Time to downshift. Yin yoga, stretching, or rest—all count.

And if you don't cycle? You still have natural rhythms: daily energy swings, seasonal patterns, stress peaks. The same principle applies: Move with your rhythm instead of against it.

### Case Study: The Perimenopause Pivot

Meet Lila, forty-four, who spent years crushing HIIT classes until she realized she was exhausted, irritable, and awake at 3 a.m. every night. She swapped half her HIIT sessions for yoga and strength training, started taking real rest days, and within a month was sleeping through the night again.

Movement didn't fix everything, but it stopped working against her body.

## Perimenopause, Cortisol, and Why Rest Days Matter

In your late thirties and forties, estrogen starts to fluctuate and cortisol gets clingy. Too much high-intensity exercise can backfire, spiking stress hormones further. That stubborn weight gain around your middle? It's often hormonal.

Rest is strategy. Rest days lower cortisol, restore sleep, and make your next workout actually work for you instead of depleting you further.

---

### EXPERT SIDEBAR:

"While cardio gets most of the spotlight, strength training, flexibility work, and mindful movement like yoga all support cardiovascular and hormonal health—especially during transitions like perimenopause. The key is consistency over intensity."

---

## Bottom Line

Community movement is one of the simplest, most powerful ways to boost mental health. It heals loneliness, balances hormones, lowers cortisol, and reminds your nervous system you're not alone.

And when you pair that social connection with movement that honors your body's natural rhythms—whether that's your menstrual cycle, your energy patterns, or your season of life—you're not just exercising. You're recalibrating your entire system.

Whether it's a barre class, a walk with a friend, or a text-thread stretch club, the magic is the same: Moving together, and moving wisely, rewires both body and brain for resilience.

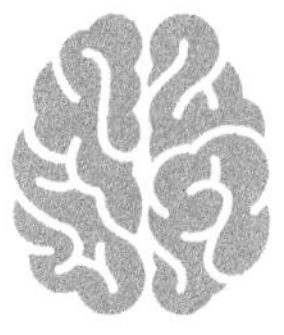



# TL;DR, DO THIS NOW, AND CLINICAL CUES

## ☑ TL;DR

- Group movement = nervous system medicine. It lowers stress, boosts mood, and fights loneliness.
- Mirror neurons make shared effort contagious. Seeing others push inspires your brain to do the same.
- Walking-and-talking is therapy in sneakers. Motion unlocks emotion.
- Movement regulates hormones: It lowers cortisol, balances estrogen/progesterone shifts, and smooths PMS/perimenopause symptoms.
- Rest days = hormonal strategy.

- Oxytocin from high-fives, hugs, and shared sweat bonds you to your people and buffers stress.

## ☑ Do This Now

- Schedule a movement date: Text one friend and set up a walk, yoga class, or "errand stroll." Even twenty minutes counts.
- Try a low-lift community hack: Join a virtual class, start a group text accountability thread, or swap a seated meeting for a "moving meeting."
- Hormone-friendly choice: If you're in a low-energy phase (PMS, perimenopause, or just exhausted), swap HIIT for stretching or Pilates. Your body will thank you.
- Add one touchpoint: High-five, fist bump, or hug someone after shared movement. Oxytocin boost = unlocked.
- Plan a rest day: Treat it like part of training, and don't skip it. Rest regulates hormones and rebuilds resilience.

## ☑ Clinical Cues

- **Oxytocin (serum, not widely available but measurable in functional labs)**

**Why it matters:** Group movement, laughter, and shared effort all raise oxytocin, the bonding hormone. Low oxytocin is linked with anxiety, loneliness, and postpartum depression. Women who feel isolated often score lower here, and movement with others is one of the fastest natural "boosters."

■ **Cortisol (a.m./p.m. or four-point saliva/urine)**

- Normal a.m.: 6–23 µg/dL with smooth taper to night
- Optimal: 10–18 µg/dL morning, <5 µg/dL evening

**Why it matters:** Moving in community lowers cortisol more effectively than solo workouts. High evening cortisol (wired, can't sleep) often softens when exercise is combined with social bonding.

■ **Heart Rate Variability (HRV, wearable or functional testing)**

- Optimal: Higher is better (varies by device).

**Why it matters:** HRV reflects parasympathetic (calm) versus sympathetic (stress) tone. Women in community classes often see HRV rise faster than with solo routines, meaning their nervous systems adapt better to stress.

■ **High-Sensitivity C-Reactive Protein (hs-CRP)**

- Normal: <3 mg/L
- Optimal: <1 mg/L

**Why it matters:** Community and connection are inflammation lowering. Women with strong social ties who also move consistently tend to show lower CRP, translating to fewer mood swings and better resilience.

■ **Endorphin/β-Endorphin (specialty functional panel)**

**Why it matters:** Not a common test, but some advanced labs measure it. Group exercise elevates endorphins more robustly than solitary movement, explaining the "post-class high" that improves mood regulation.

## ☑ Moving On

We've learned that while exercise is good, exercising in community is even better. In Part 4, we'll dive deeper into the benefits of friendship, exploring how meaningful, intentional community can be one of the most effective tools for mental health and healing. Whom you move with matters. Whom you let into your inner circle matters more. But don't worry. We'll get into the science of boundaries, chosen family, and emotional safety soon. For now, grab a buddy, lace up your sneakers, and get moving. Because healing doesn't have to be lonely. And sometimes, the fastest way to a better mood is shared sweat and silly playlists.

# PART 3 RECAP: MOVE YOUR BODY; MOVE YOUR MIND

So, what have we learned in Part 3? That movement is medicine: maintenance for your brain, your hormones, and your nervous system. Not punishment. Not a chore.

Here's the highlight reel:

- Your body evolved to move, not to sit still like a decorative throw pillow. Sedentary stress is real, and your brain knows it.
- Movement flips ancient switches in your biology, releasing endorphins, dopamine, serotonin, GABA, and BDNF, magical molecules that literally rewire your mood and resilience.
- Find movement that feels good: dancing in your kitchen, walking with a friend, stretching before bed.
- Micromovements count. Rolling your shoulders or walking to grab the mail tells your nervous system "Hey, we're safe. We're thriving."
- Group movement? That's a two-for-one deal: sweat plus connection. It heals your brain chemistry and bonds you to others.
- Your hormones (yes, even the messy ones) love movement. Whether it's PMS, perimenopause, or cortisol chaos, exercise helps smooth the ride.
- Rest days are hormonal strategy and nervous system support.

The big takeaway? Move in ways that remind your brain and body you're alive, safe, and still capable of joy.

## Movement → Connection

Movement is a load capacity restoration tool. When you move your body, you're actively metabolizing stress hormones, regulating cortisol, and signaling safety to your nervous system.

Every walk, dance session, or yoga class increases your capacity to handle emotional and cognitive demands. Sedentary living keeps your nervous system locked in a low-capacity state where even small stressors feel overwhelming. Think of movement as actively charging your battery: It increases mitochondrial function (more cellular energy), improves insulin sensitivity (stable blood sugar equals stable mood), enhances BDNF production (brain repair), and downregulates your stress response. When your Clinical Cues include brain fog after sitting, anxiety that eases with walking, or mood crashes when you skip movement, your body is telling you: Movement is medicine. And unlike supplements, you can't take too much of it.

# PART 4

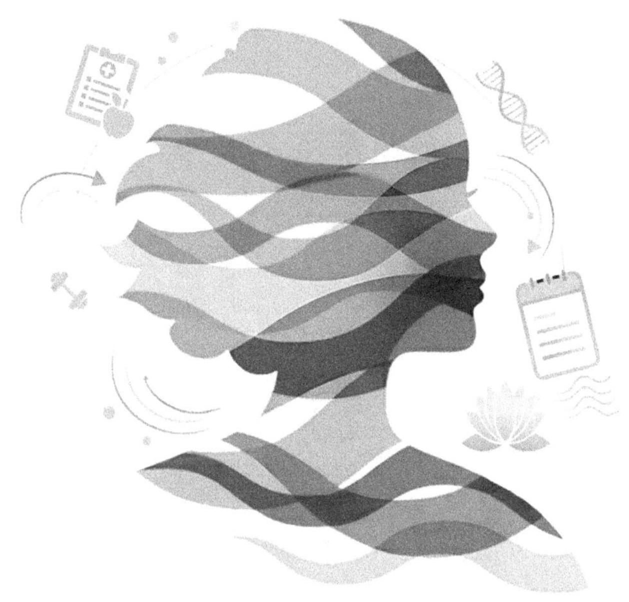

## BECAUSE EVEN YOUR BRAIN NEEDS A GROUP CHAT

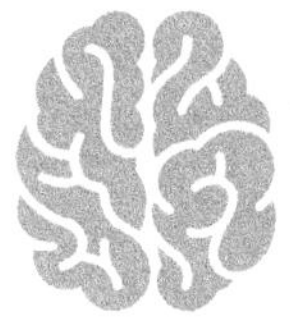

# CHAPTER 15

# THE LONELINESS EPIDEMIC

Your brain wasn't built to go it alone. It evolved in tribes, in tight-knit communities where survival meant closeness. Now? We're social creatures trapped in isolated routines, and our nervous systems are paying the price.

Loneliness goes deeper than missing weekend plans or half-hearted "HBD" texts from friends who ghosted you in 2019. It's a full-blown health crisis, and science is finally catching up to what your nervous system has known for years: Isolation hurts.

When I was a kid in the nineties, I knew every house on the block. I played outside until the streetlights came on, knocked on doors without warning, and shared long stretches of real eye contact and laughter with every kid I knew. These days, connection looks different.

Loneliness is a full-body physiological event. Connection is medicine: science-backed, nervous system–soothing, essential.

## So, What Is Loneliness, Anyway?

Loneliness is the distress that comes from having fewer quality relationships than you desire.

Your body on loneliness:

- Increased cortisol
- Elevated inflammatory markers (CRP, IL-6)
- Higher anxiety and depression risk
- Poorer sleep quality
- Cognitive decline

A landmark study by Holt-Lunstad et al. (2015) found that loneliness increases the risk of premature death by 26%, making it as deadly as smoking fifteen cigarettes a day. In 2023, the US Surgeon General declared loneliness a public health epidemic.

This is biochemistry, not poetry.

## Alone Versus Lonely: Your Body Knows the Difference

There's a critical distinction between being alone and being lonely.

- Alone: Chosen, restorative, empowering. Boosts creativity and focus. Stress hormones drop.

- Lonely: Unwanted, heavy. A feeling of restlessness and emotional invisibility. Cortisol and inflammation spike.

Your body knows the difference. Solitude can be medicine. Loneliness is a stressor.

You don't need *more* people; you need the *right* people.

## Your Immune System Needs Friends

Your immune system, that thing you've been trying to support with zinc gummies and hand sanitizer, actually gets a boost from regular, positive social interaction.

A landmark study from Carnegie Mellon University [Cohen et al. (1997)] found that people with diverse, supportive social ties were less likely to develop colds after being exposed to a virus. You read that right: Hugging your friend could make you less likely to get sick.

Meanwhile, social isolation triggers inflammation and hormonal imbalance that weakens immune response. Being disconnected is a literal stressor, and your body takes it very seriously.

## Anxiety, Cortisol, and Lonely Brain Chemistry

Ever notice how your nervous system slows its roll after a heart-to-heart with someone who gets you? That's biochemistry at work.

Positive social interaction:

- Reduces cortisol, your stress hormone
- Activates oxytocin, the bonding hormone that says, "You're safe here."

A 2014 meta-analysis in *Personality and Social Psychology Review* found strong links between social support and reduced anxiety and depression symptoms. Connection literally downregulates your stress response like a deep exhale wrapped in human presence.

## Brain Gains from Being Social

Social interaction, especially the emotionally meaningful kind improves memory and cognitive function, particularly as we age.

Studies from Harvard and the Rush Alzheimer's Disease Center show seniors with frequent social contact maintain better cognitive health and are at reduced risk of dementia.

Translation: Talking to your neighbor about her cats is a mental workout with a side of community.

## Your Brain on Friendship (and Oxytocin)

Community literally changes what's happening in your brain.

Here's how time with people you love changes the chemistry between your ears:

- Oxytocin, the "cuddle hormone," is released for safety, trust, and stress regulation.
- Dopamine, serotonin, and endogenous opioids flood your system, improving mood and motivation and relieving pain.
- Mirror neurons sync your emotions to others; calm borrows calm.

Emotional states ripple through relationships. Our nervous systems sync more than we realize. When we're around people who feel grounded, hopeful, or steady, our bodies often borrow some of that regulation. And on the hard days, we offer it back.

The point isn't to avoid anyone who's struggling. Humans are designed to co-carry stress. The real takeaway is that connection is literally a biological exchange: We regulate each other, we soften each other, and sometimes we steady each other just by being there.

We don't need perfect people around us. We just need people who show up. That's how nervous systems stay sane.

## Connection as Medicine: The Research

### Social Prescribing: Friendship, but Make It Medical

In the UK and Australia, doctors are literally writing prescriptions for connection: join clubs, volunteer, attend group walks, participate in mutual aid networks.

A 2022 *British Medical Journal* report found that social prescribing improved mental well-being, reduced GP visits, and increased life satisfaction. Friendship is clinical.

### Volunteering: The Unexpected Longevity Benefit

Volunteering boosts self-esteem, strengthens purpose, and increases dopamine and endorphins. According to a study published in *Health Psychology* [Konrath et al. (2012)], people who volunteer regularly have a 22% lower risk of dying over four years.

Because altruistic volunteering lights up reward circuits, strengthens social bonds, and reinforces safety signaling, your body reads it as connection, not isolation, which is one of the most protective biological states we can be in.

> ### Case Study: Maya's Walking Group
>
> Meet Maya, forty-two. Corporate lawyer, queen of unread Slack notifications, and part-time DoorDash addict. For years, her nights ended with Netflix autoplay and wine. Not because she loved solitude, but because she was too exhausted to reach out.
>
> One Saturday, she reluctantly joined a neighborhood walking group, mostly because her doctor side-eyed her blood pressure.
>
> Within two weeks, her evenings looked different: laughter instead of silence, a shared pace instead of scrolling alone.
>
> She didn't suddenly become extroverted. She just remembered what her nervous system had been begging for: connection.
>
> Maya didn't fix her whole life. But she went from "Fine, I'll walk" to "I actually look forward to this." That's nervous system medicine.

## Digital Connection Versus Real Connection

Social media gives us the illusion of intimacy, but likes and follows don't light up the same neural pathways that activate when we're face-to-face. [Twenge et al. (2017)]

Those in-person social cues—vocal tone, microexpressions, subtle body language—are processed through brain regions tied to safety, reward, and belonging. They trigger oxytocin, soothe the amygdala, and reinforce the sense that we're part of a tribe.

In contrast, digital connection without depth tends to bypass those circuits. It feels stimulating, but not regulating. We scroll more and bond less. Our brains stay slightly guarded, slightly lonely, slightly wired for threat.

But let's not lose our nuance. Online connection isn't bad. A late-night voice memo from your best friend, a heartfelt FaceTime call, or a real emotional exchange over text can still hit your oxytocin receptors. The difference is intention and depth.

Passive scrolling is isolation. Intentional sharing is medicine.

## COVID-19: The Great Social Disconnect

And then came 2020.

Social distancing kept us safe from a virus, but it gutted our connection infrastructure. Overnight, we lost casual interactions: the coffee shop regulars, the gym friends, the coworker lunch breaks, the spontaneous hugs. The fabric of everyday connection unraveled.

In 2021, *The Lancet* reported a global 25% spike in anxiety and depression, with social isolation identified as a major culprit. But the numbers don't capture what it felt like: the bone-deep loneliness of staring at screens all day, the fatigue of Zoom calls that somehow felt more draining than real conversation, the quiet desperation of months without physical touch.

We adapted. We had to. Virtual happy hours, socially distanced walks, porch visits. These workarounds fell short of what our nervous systems were wired for: proximity, physical presence, the neurobiological reassurance of being in the same room.

## The Lingering Effects

Even as the acute phase of the pandemic ended, the social damage persisted. Many of us lost the habit of reaching out. Social muscles atrophied. Anxiety around gathering increased. We got used to isolation, not because we preferred it, but because reentering felt overwhelming.

Research from the American Psychological Association found that even after restrictions lifted, rates of loneliness remained elevated, particularly among young adults and women. The pandemic didn't just isolate us temporarily; it rewired our social patterns, and many of us are still trying to find our way back.

## What We Lost (And What We're Rebuilding)

The pandemic forced us to realize how much of our connection was passive and ambient; the brief conversations, the body language across a conference table, the casual physical proximity that signaled safety to our nervous systems.

Now, connection requires more intention. We can't rely on default social infrastructure. We have to actively build it: Schedule the coffee dates, plan the walks, text first even when it feels awkward.

The good news? Intentional connection, when we actually show up for it, can be deeper and more nourishing than the passive variety we lost. We're learning to be more deliberate about who we spend time with and how. That's not a consolation prize. That's an evolution.

## Why Women Feel Loneliness Differently

Women are often told that needing people makes us "clingy" or "too emotional," even though research shows that women are consistently more sensitive to changes in social support than men. [Hawkley and Cacioppo (2010); Umberson et al. (1996)]

Add in caregiving roles, career pressures, and the cultural expectation to be hyper-independent, and it makes sense that many women end up downplaying their need for connection.

But biology doesn't care about those narratives. Across multiple studies, social connection has a stronger effect on women's emotional well-being, stress physiology, and mental health than it does for men. [Hall (2011); Park (2021)]

## The Science

Sex-specific oxytocin responses: Women show stronger increases in oxytocin when facing interpersonal stress or psychological distress than men, potentially mediated by sex hormones.

Differential neural effects: In human imaging studies, oxytocin alters amygdala activity differently in men than in women. For women, exposure to social praise (versus criticism) increased positive social perception under oxytocin, while in men it didn't follow the same pattern. [Gao et al., (2016)]

Gendered stress-response patterns: In stress experiments where participants faced social stress or isolation, women showed elevated cortisol reactions, whereas men were more reactive under "challenge/achievement" stress.

Your nervous system still needs safe, consistent connection. Period.

## What You Can Do

Connection is your medicine, and it doesn't have to be hard to access. Here are some simple ideas to win yourself some cozy connected brain chemistry:

Reach out: one text, one walk, one check-in. Connection doesn't require a full-blown hangout or a three-hour dinner. One intentional moment of contact is enough to nudge your oxytocin system and soften cortisol. Send a warm check-in text. Invite someone on a simple walk. Share a thought, a win, or even a hard moment. Microconnection counts.

Be honest: say, "I'm lonely." (Someone else probably is too.) Loneliness thrives in silence. Naming how you feel gives someone else permission to tell the truth too. Instead of performing "busy" or "fine," lead with vulnerability. Let the people you trust know you want more warmth, more conversation, more shared moments.

Give it a rhythm. Schedule it. Make it predictable. Monthly dinner with the same friend group. A recurring Sunday voice-memo catch-up. A weekly meme exchange thread with a sibling or best friend. First-Friday coffee dates. A same-time daily text check-in. All count. Predictable, repeated social contact cues safety to the nervous system, removing pressure, awkwardness, and overthinking, so connection runs on autopilot.

Move together: dance classes, group walks, clubs. Shared movement bonds people faster than small talk. Synchrony, walking at the same pace, doing the same steps, following the same rhythm literally blends nervous systems. It boosts endorphins, softens stress hormones, and makes strangers feel familiar.

Therapy: Break the feedback loop. When isolation, stress, or old relational wounds start looping, therapy creates a safe structure for connection, reflection, and emotional recalibration. Having one consistent, attuned relationship, even professionally, reminds the brain that connection can be secure, nonjudgmental, and steady. It's not just talk. It's nervous system corrective experience.

## Microcheck Ritual: The Connection Pulse

Once a week, pause and ask yourself:

- When's the last time I felt truly connected?
- Who gives me energy when I'm around them?
- Who drains me and why am I still giving them access?

Your body is giving you live feedback.

## Bottom Line

You are not built for isolation. Your brain, your immune system, your stress response, all of them function better when you're connected to people who see you, hear you, and show up consistently.

Connection isn't a luxury. It's a biological necessity. The good news? You just need a few people who feel safe, a few rituals that create rhythm, and the willingness to reach out even when it feels vulnerable.

Your nervous system will thank you.

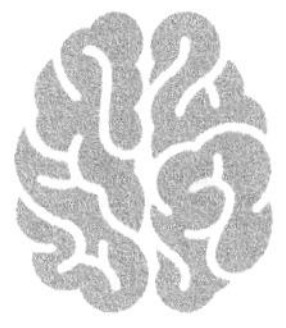



# TL;DR, DO THIS NOW, AND CLINICAL CUES

## ☑ TL;DR

- Loneliness is a health risk as serious as smoking.
- Social interaction boosts immunity, lowers stress hormones, and protects memory.
- Connection releases oxytocin, dopamine, and serotonin, literal medicine.
- Quality matters more than quantity: the *right* people regulate your nervous system.
- For women especially, needing people reflects biological strength.

## ☑ Do This Now

- Send one genuine check-in text or voice memo today.
- Schedule one ritual of connection, like a walk, dinner, or call.
- Try the "Connection Pulse" questions to audit your social circle.

## ☑ Clinical Cues

### ▪ High-Sensitivity C-Reactive Protein (hs-CRP)

- Normal: <3 mg/L
- Optimal: <1 mg/L

**Why it matters:** Loneliness is inflammatory, literally. Women who feel chronically disconnected often show elevated CRP, which links to depression, cardiovascular disease, and cognitive decline.

### ▪ TNF-α and IL-1β (cytokines, specialty labs)

**Why it matters:** Chronic stress and poor diet raise these. They're linked to depression, "sickness behavior," and brain fog.

### ▪ Cortisol (four-point diurnal curve)

- Normal a.m.: 6–23 µg/dL, tapering by evening
- Optimal: Strong a.m. rise, <5 µg/dL at night

**Why it matters:** Loneliness dysregulates cortisol rhythms. Instead of the energizing morning spike, women often get a flat curve → fatigue, poor sleep, increased anxiety.

### ▪ Heart Rate Variability (HRV)

- Optimal: Higher is better for resilience (varies by device).

**Why it matters:** Loneliness tanks HRV, leaving the nervous system stuck in fight-or-flight mode. Group connection, touch, and belonging improve HRV, translating to emotional stability and lower stress reactivity.

### ▪ Lipid Panel (total cholesterol, LDL, HDL, triglycerides)

**Why it matters:** Chronic social isolation correlates with higher LDL and triglycerides. Women in midlife often chalk this up to aging, when in reality disconnection is driving silent metabolic changes.

## ☑ Moving On

Your nervous system needs connection, not crowds. It needs resonance, not noise. Start with one person who helps you feel safe, seen, and steady. That's medicine. In the next chapter, we'll take a look at the social science behind building the kind of community you and your nervous system need and how to put that science to work.

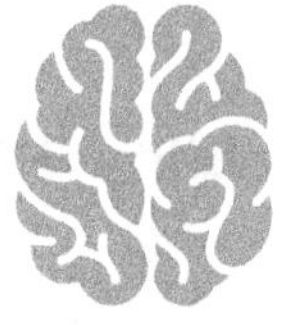



# QUALITY OVER QUANTITY (BECAUSE YOU DON'T NEED THIRTY-SEVEN BEST FRIENDS)

Can we be real for a sec? Somewhere along the way, society convinced us that having a massive social circle is the gold standard of emotional success. That what we all need is Instagram followers, group chats that are somehow always muted, and a "Catch up soon!" loop with half the people you went to college with. The myth? That being good with people means knowing everyone, getting invited to everything, and showing up with the emotional stamina of a TED Talk speaker on espresso.

But here's the truth bomb your nervous system has been waiting for: Having a few deeply connected, emotionally safe relationships will always outweigh having thirty-seven brunch friends and zero real ones.

And here's where boundaries come in. You don't have to keep every connection on life support just because you shared a dorm room once. Emotional energy is not infinite, and pretending otherwise is the fastest way to land in exhaustion disguised as social success.

## Your Brain's Limits: Dunbar's Number

Zoom out and look at your social life through a brain lens for a minute. Yes, your brain craves people, and it's wired for connection, but it also has limits. Enter Dunbar's number, a theory proposed by British anthropologist Robin Dunbar, suggesting that humans can realistically maintain about 150 social relationships at once. And here's the catch: That number includes the outer-ring people too. Your coworker's baby-shower friend, your ex-roommate's new boyfriend, and the neighbor you wave to but don't actually know. When it comes to *real intimacy,* the kind that softens your nervous system and actually makes your life better, you're looking at five. Maybe even three on a bad week. That's your true ride-or-die tier, and frankly, that's plenty.

Depth matters more than numbers when it comes to relationships that nourish you. Emotional bandwidth is like a Jenga tower: Each stressor pulls a block. Keep stacking, and eventually, the whole thing wobbles.

## Green Flags Versus Red Flags

Not sure who belongs in your inner circle? Use your body as the barometer. Here's your quick cheat sheet.

*Green Flags*

- You feel lighter after talking.
- They respect your boundaries without a guilt trip.
- They celebrate your wins without competition.
- You can ugly-cry and not apologize after.

*Red Flags*

- You brace yourself before texting back.
- Conversations feel like performance or competition.
- You leave drained, not filled.
- Your body tenses at the thought of seeing them.

Run this check on any relationship in your life that you're wondering about. The answers will tell you everything.

## A Micro Story: Brunch with a Side of Burnout

I knew I needed a reset when I walked out of brunch more tired than I had walked in, like I'd just survived an emotional CrossFit class I never signed up for. The conversation was all humble brags, veiled digs, and obligatory selfies. I got home, dropped onto the couch, and thought, *If this is friendship, my nervous system is doomed.* That was the day I realized this: If the vibe is dread before and depletion after, walk away.

So I did something radical for a chronic people pleaser: I paused those friendships. Not with drama or a speech. Just space. I stopped forcing brunches that left me buzzing with cortisol, and paid attention to who I actually felt safe with. It took a couple months, but my body noticed long before my brain did. I started feeling lighter after conversations instead of depleted. Shared laughter lingered. Silence didn't feel like rejection. That's when I knew that real connection is the kind that regulates your nervous system, not wrecks it.

## Attachment Styles and Why They Matter

Here's the science-y sidenote your inner psych nerd will love: The way you connect with others often traces back to attachment theory, pioneered by John Bowlby and expanded by Mary Ainsworth. More recently, books like *Attached* by Amir Levine and Rachel S.F. Heller and *The Polyvagal Theory* by Stephen W. Porges have connected the dots between attachment patterns and nervous system regulation. Here's the top-line info you need to know:

- Secure attachment: These relationships feel safe. Your nervous system settles. Stress hormones drop. You can show up authentically without strategizing every word.
- Anxious attachment: Relationships feel unpredictable. You might feel hypervigilant, scanning for rejection. Your nervous system hovers in fight-or-flight mode.

- Avoidant attachment: Intimacy feels suffocating. You pull away to self-regulate, but your nervous system stays on guard.
- Disorganized attachment: A mix of anxious and avoidant. Your nervous system ricochets between craving closeness and fearing it.

When you build secure, high-quality friendships, you're retraining your nervous system to rest, repair, and thrive in connection.

## The Physiology of Feeling Safe

Emotionally safe relationships do more than feel good. They regulate your nervous system at a physiological level. Stress hormones drop. Immune function improves. Your body shifts from fight-or-flight into rest-and-digest mode.

In the Harvard Study of Adult Development, higher relationship warmth at midlife predicted healthier cardiovascular profiles decades later, including lower ambulatory blood pressure and reduced physiological stress burden. [Waldinger, Schulz, et al. (2015)] The study followed adults across their lifespan and found that the quality of intimate relationships at age fifty was a stronger predictor of healthy aging than cholesterol, income, or medical history. In other words: Stable, trusting connection functions as a long-range buffer against the wear-and-tear mechanisms that drive disease.

## The Friendship Audit

So how do you start pruning and protecting your energy? Try this simple ritual once or twice a year:

1. Write down the names of your ten to fifteen closest connections.
2. For each name on the list, ask yourself:
    a. Do I feel lighter or heavier after spending time with them?
    b. Can I show up messy, or do I feel like I need to perform?
    c. Do they respect my boundaries or negotiate them?
    d. Have I been overgenerous to this person?
3. Circle your "green flag" people. Put stars by the ones you want to nurture more.
4. For the "red flag" folks? Release, redefine, or at least reduce your investment.

Remember: Boundaries are not walls. They're bridges to healthier connection. They let the right people in and keep your energy safe from the wrong ones.

## The Permission Slip You Needed

You're allowed to prioritize fewer, deeper relationships. You're allowed to say no to surface-level socializing that leaves you feeling hollow. You're allowed to prune your circle down to the roots and rebuild with intention. Wanting peace means you're practicing self-respect.

Being known matters more than being liked.

No glittery group photo will ever compete with the quiet, steady safety of being truly seen and loved. The real magic lives in protecting the connections that regulate your nervous system and remind you who you are.

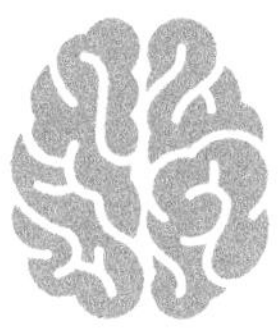



# TL;DR, DO THIS NOW, AND CLINICAL CUES

## ☑ TL;DR

- Your nervous system cares about safety in your closest relationships, not follower counts.
- Relationship quality predicts happiness and health more than quantity.
- Attachment styles (secure, anxious, avoidant, disorganized) inform how your body responds to connection, and knowing about your attachment style can help you work on becoming more secure.
- Secure relationships regulate your nervous system.
- Green flags: You feel lighter, safe, and fully yourself.

- Red flags: You feel tension, self-monitoring, dread, or the bone-deep fatigue that hits after spending time together. Sometimes your body registers the drain before your mind can name why. Pay attention to that.
- A handful of secure, emotionally safe friendships is worth infinitely more than thirty-seven brunch friends who drain you.

## ☑ Do This Now

1. Run a friendship audit: Write down the names of your ten to fifteen closest connections. Circle the ones who make you feel safe, supported, and seen. Put stars next to the ones you want to nurture more.
2. Spot your flags: Notice who makes your shoulders drop (green flag) versus who makes your stomach clench (red flag). Adjust your energy accordingly.
3. Check your attachment lens: Ask yourself "Do I feel calm, anxious, avoidant, or mixed in this relationship?" Seek out connections that support secure attachment and nervous system regulation.
4. Invest in depth, not volume: Prioritize quality time with your gold-tier people. That's nervous system medicine, not just socializing.

## ☑ Clinical Cues

### ▨ Oxytocin (serum or urine, specialty test)

**Why it matters:** Deep, safe relationships raise oxytocin, the "bonding hormone." Low levels are linked to anxiety, postpartum mood struggles, and difficulty feeling connected. Having thirty acquaintances won't raise oxytocin the way two close friends will.

### ▨ Cortisol (four-point diurnal curve)

- Normal a.m.: 6–23 µg/dL tapering into evening
- Optimal: Strong morning rise, <5 µg/dL at night

**Why it matters:** Women with solid social support have healthier cortisol rhythms. Shallow or toxic connections leave cortisol flat or erratic, showing up as fatigue, irritability, and poor sleep.

### ▨ Heart Rate Variability (HRV, wearable or functional test)

- Optimal: Higher is better (device-specific range).

**Why it matters:** HRV reflects nervous system safety. Women with even one secure, high-quality bond show higher HRV than women with dozens of surface-level friendships. High HRV = resilience and emotional regulation.

### ▩ Interleukin-6 (IL-6, cytokine, specialty)

**Why it matters:** This inflammation marker spikes in toxic relationships. It's not just loneliness that inflames you; being in the wrong crowd can be just as damaging, leading to anxiety, autoimmune flare-ups, and depressive symptoms.

**Sex Hormone Binding Globulin (SHBG, serum)**

- Normal: 18–144 nmol/L (women, varies by lab)
- Optimal: Mid-range, context-specific

**Why it matters:** Chronic toxic stress lowers SHBG, skewing estrogen and testosterone balance. Women often feel this as PMS chaos, hormonal acne, or midlife metabolic struggles. High-quality connections buffer stress and keep SHBG in a healthier range.

## ☑ Moving On

We've seen how connection keeps us regulated and how when it comes to relationships, our nervous systems will always put quality over quantity. Let's summarize everything we've learned in Part 4, before making friends with our own minds in Part 5.

# PART 4 RECAP: CONNECTION IS LITERALLY MEDICINE

Loneliness is a full-on health hazard, not just a sad Saturday night. When you're disconnected, your body feels bad and functions worse. Cortisol? Through the roof. Inflammation? Up like it's trying to make a statement. Your immune system? Acting like it forgot how to defend you. Studies [hello, Holt-Lunstad et al. (2015)] show that chronic loneliness raises your risk of premature death by 26%. That's the same as smoking fifteen cigarettes a day. And no one's glamorizing that habit anymore.

Now, flip the script: Connection is literal medicine. We're talking about your body's DIY pharmacy kicking into high gear. Oxytocin (trust, bonding), dopamine (motivation, pleasure), serotonin (mood stability), endogenous opioids (pain relief) and all those delicious neurochemicals flow when you're with people who get you. One good laugh, one tight hug, one deep conversation, and boom! Your nervous system exhales like it's been holding its breath for years.

It's important to note that loneliness triggers your stress response, plain and simple. Evolution wired us to thrive in tribes. Alone = vulnerable. Vulnerable = danger. That's why your body treats loneliness like a real, physical threat. Elevated cortisol, higher inflammation, poor sleep, even cognitive decline, the receipts are in. This affects survival, not just mood.

During COVID-19, we all got a taste of this. Social distancing was crucial, but it didn't come without a cost. Anxiety, depression, a

25% global increase in mental health disorders [(2021) *The Lancet*], all fueled by isolation. Suddenly, that Zoom call didn't quite replace a hug, did it? Back in the nineties, connection meant knocking on your friend's door, playing outside until the streetlights came on, and fighting over who got the last Capri-Sun. Now? Social media's giving us the illusion of intimacy, but our brains aren't fooled. Likes don't replace laughter. Stories don't replace storytelling. More screen time is consistently linked with increased loneliness, lower psychological well-being, and poorer social fulfillment in teens, especially compared with face-to-face connection. [Twenge and Campbell, (2018)] Large cohort follow-up data showed the same trend after widespread smartphone adoption in 2012. [Twenge, Haidt, Joiner, and Campbell (2020)] We're more "connected" than ever, but somehow, we're lonelier too.

## Your Brain Was Built to Belong

Rejection lights up the same neural circuits as physical pain, particularly the dorsal anterior cingulate cortex. [Eisenberger, Lieberman, and Williams (2003)] The opposite is also true: Secure social connection activates parasympathetic pathways that lower heart rate, cortisol, and inflammation. Strong, consistent relationships are literally survival mechanisms. A large meta-analysis of 148 studies found that robust social ties predict a 50% increase in survival, comparable to quitting smoking. [Holt-Lunstad, Smith, and Layton (2010)]

Volunteering, especially when motivated by genuine care for others, is associated with a roughly 22% reduction in mortality.

[Okun, Yeung, and Brown (2013)] And physicians are now using "social prescribing," structured referrals to community groups, volunteering, movement classes, arts programs, and connection-based environments because it reliably improves mental health outcomes and reduces clinical burden, including GP visits and anxiety symptoms. [Bickerdike et al. (2017)]

## Alone Versus Lonely: Know the Difference

Being alone? That's chosen solitude, and it's actually good for you. It fuels creativity, helps you regulate emotions, and gives your nervous system a breather. It's sipping coffee in silence, walking without earbuds, or finally finishing a book without interruptions.

Feeling lonely? That's craving connection and not finding it. It's being in a room full of people and still feeling unseen. It's your brain whispering, "We need someone." And if ignored, it becomes chronic, interfering with your mood, focus, and physical health. Safe to say, connection is a necessity.

### Here's What You Can Actually Do About It

- **Reach out:** One phone call beats twenty doomscroll texts. Voice carries tone, warmth, and regulation cues your nervous system can't get from a screen. Call a friend while folding laundry. Leave a voice memo instead of a heart emoji. Human sounds > typed blurbs.
- **Create rituals of connection:** Predictable routines calm the nervous system. Schedule monthly dinners with the same people, Sunday morning coffee walks, or a standing "Wednesday

evening check-in" with someone you trust. When connection has a rhythm, no one has to wonder if they're intruding or "needy." The structure holds the closeness.

- **Move with others:** Join a class, take a walk with a friend, sign up for a volunteer shift, or go to a community workout. Movement synchronizes breath, gait, and mirror neurons, which is nature's fastest way to reduce stress and build intimacy. Bodies bonding in space beats isolation behind screens.

- **Talk honestly:** Loneliness shrinks when someone says, "Me too." Name what's real. Skip the performance. Authenticity is a biochemical invitation: Truth triggers oxytocin, eye contact boosts dopamine, and mutual vulnerability regulates stress responses. Honesty is nervous system medicine.

Connection is a biological necessity that directly impacts your load capacity. When you're isolated, your nervous system treats it as a threat, keeping cortisol elevated, inflammation higher, and your capacity to regulate emotions significantly reduced. This is why loneliness feels physically exhausting: Your body is burning through capacity just managing the physiological stress of disconnection. Co-regulation (the nervous system phenomenon where proximity to safe others literally calms your biology) is one of the most powerful capacity-restoration tools available.

When you're in the presence of someone whose nervous system is regulated, yours follows. Your Clinical Cues for connection-related load depletion include: feeling emotionally raw when alone for too long, noticing you think more clearly after meaningful conversation, or experiencing physical relief (deeper breathing, relaxed shoulders) in safe company. Quality relationships measurably increase your capacity to handle everything else in your life. Beyoncé doesn't run her empire alone. Neither should you. You can be powerful and connected. Strong and supported.

## Quick Gut Check: Are You Connection Deprived or Co-Regulated?

Answer honestly; your nervous system will know if you're lying.

1. When something great (or terrible) happens, whom do you tell first?

   A. I have a go-to person or two.

   B. I hesitate, then maybe post something vague online.

   C. I bottle it up or talk to my plants (they're great listeners).

2. After hanging out with people, how do you usually feel?

   A. Seen, lighter, like myself again.

   B. Neutral, like I ticked off a task.

   C. Emotionally jet-lagged and in need of a nap.

3. How often do you experience genuine, eye contact–level connection (not screen-to-screen)?

   A. Weekly or more often.

   B. Maybe monthly?

   C. What is eye contact again?

4. When you're overwhelmed, who helps you co-regulate?

   A. I've got a few people I can fully fall apart with.

   B. I have people, but I don't always reach out.

   C. I don't really feel like I can lean on anyone.

5.  Do your current relationships feel emotionally safe?

    A. Yes, they're my recharge stations.

    B. Somewhat, depends on the day.

    C. Not really, I'm constantly performing or holding back.

## Your Nervous System Scorecard

- Mostly As: You're co-regulated and connected. You've built a community that fuels you. Keep tending to it like your emotional garden.
- Mostly Bs: You're connection aware but a little undernourished. Time to initiate, reach out, and deepen your bonds. Go beyond "How are you?"
- Mostly Cs: Your connection tank is running on fumes. This isn't an accusation; it's a gentle nudge. Prioritize small, safe steps toward intimacy. You don't need ten people. Start with one.

## Challenge

Text someone right now and tell them you appreciate them. Not someday. Not later. Now. The science says your brain, and theirs, will thank you.

You need the right people, not more people. Quality over quantity, always. Whether it's one "ride or die" or a handful of solid souls, connection is how you heal, grow, and thrive.

So call the friend. Say yes to the dinner invite. Sit across from someone, and let your nervous systems talk to each other.

Face-to-face connection provides synchronized breath, vocal tone, laughter, eye contact, and safety cues. Texting doesn't. In one fMRI study, emotional support over text did *not* reduce threat-response in the brain, but hearing the voice of someone trusted did. Digital contact acknowledges you. Real-time presence regulates you.

Your biology isn't asking for more notifications. It's asking for proximity strong enough to lower cortisol and raise oxytocin. And you? You deserve connection that helps your system settle, your heart rate drop, and your body finally exhale.

Connection you can *feel*.

# PART 5

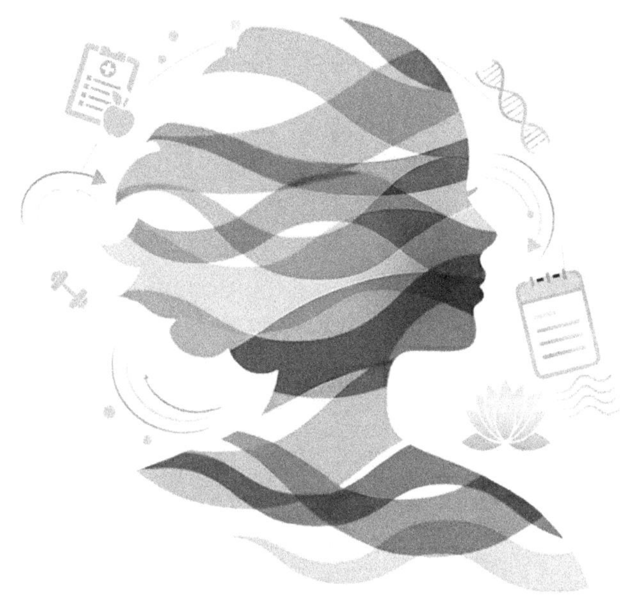

# MIND OVER MATTER (AND MOOD): THE CASE FOR MINDFULNESS IN A CHAOTIC WORLD

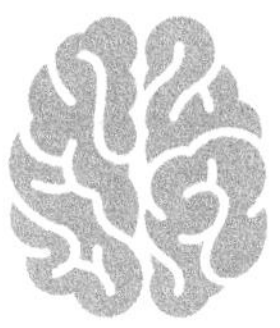



# WAIT, IS THIS A CULT?

Let's clear the air: Mindfulness isn't a cult. Yes, wellness culture has hijacked it and stuffed it into apps, retreats, and overpriced candles. Yes, influencers with hours to spare make it look like you need a crystal collection, a meditation corner with perfect natural lighting, and zero kids screaming in the background to participate. Mindfulness is about awareness and choice. It encourages critical thinking, self-inquiry, and independence—the exact opposite of cult dynamics.

Scientifically, mindfulness strengthens the prefrontal cortex, your brain's executive control center responsible for decision-making, emotional regulation, and cognitive flexibility. [Tang et al. (2007)] You're training your brain to stop reacting like Anger from *Inside Out* and start pausing before you respond. (Side note: If you haven't watched that movie, do it. It's genuinely one of the best explanations of emotional regulation ever made.

Mindfulness teaches you to question your own reactions and choose better ones.

## Mindfulness: The Actual Definition

At its core, mindfulness is simply showing up. Fully. Intentionally. Without instantly spiraling into judgment, panic, or a mental to-do list.

Instead of trying to empty your mind, you simply notice:

- The breath in your lungs
- The thought you're looping
- The jaw you've been clenching since 9 a.m.

It's the mental equivalent of turning down the blaring radio so you can hear yourself think. You just need one breath and then another.

## Real People, Real Brains: The Samantha Story

Samantha was a lawyer running on adrenaline and chaos. Sleep-deprived and constantly on edge. When her therapist suggested mindfulness meditation, her answer was: "I don't have time to sit around and breathe."

But desperation opened the door. She started with five minutes of breathwork in her car before work. Weeks later, she wasn't snapping at colleagues, sobbing in the shower, or waking up at 3 a.m. thinking about email.

Science explains why: mindfulness reduces symptoms of

anxiety, depression, and stress, while improving emotional regulation. [Khoury et al. (2013); Goyal et al. (2014)] Brain scans even show structural changes: a regular mindfulness practice shrinks the amygdala (fear center) while strengthening the prefrontal cortex (decision-making hub). [Hölzel et al. (2011)]

This is mental weight training backed by neuroscience.

## The Nervous System Connection (Polyvagal Edition)

Mindfulness helps regulate your nervous system. Stephen Porges's polyvagal theory shows that our brains are constantly scanning our surroundings for cues of danger or safety. This process is automatic and unconscious. When our nervous system detects threat, it keeps us in fight, flight, or freeze mode.

Mindfulness cues the parasympathetic nervous system (the body's rest-and-digest mode), sending the message "You're safe. You can stand down."

That's why a single breath, taken with intention, can drop your heart rate, loosen your muscles, and unclench your gut. This is vagal tone regulation, not magic.

## Another Everyday Example: Mindfulness Without Meditating

Take Marcus, a single dad of two who thought mindfulness was "for yoga moms with crystals." His entry point? Doing dishes.

Instead of zoning out or rushing, he started focusing on the warm water, the weight of each plate, the smell of the soap. His breathing slowed. His shoulders dropped. That five-minute ritual became his reset button. No app. Just presence.

## Everyday Mindfulness Hacks (That Don't Require a Retreat)

If you want to train your nervous system to self-regulate in real time, try sprinkling the following micropractices into your day.

- Coffee pause: Before the first sip, notice the warmth, the aroma, the anticipation. Then drink.
- Stoplight reset: Take three deep breaths while waiting at a red light.
- Phone rule: Before unlocking your phone, ask, "What am I here for?"
- Shower check-in: Feel the water, notice your breath, let your mind clear.
- Two-breath email: Before hitting send, take two slow breaths. Respond; don't react.

## Myth Versus Reality: Mindfulness Edition

Myth: You have to clear your mind.
*Reality: You're noticing thoughts, not erasing them.*

Myth: It requires hours of silence.
*Reality: Even sixty seconds of presence counts.*

Myth: It's spiritual nonsense.
*Reality: Decades of neuroscience back it up.*

Myth: It makes you passive.
*Reality: It strengthens focus and resilience.*

## Why Mindfulness Now?

We live in a burnout culture: constant notifications, endless pressure to perform, and the toxic badge of "doing it all." The World Health Organization recognizes burnout as a legit syndrome. Studies link overwork to stroke, heart disease, and reduced lifespan. [WHO (2019); Pega et al. (2021)]

Mindfulness interrupts the chaos loop, no one way ticket to the moon required. It's how you reclaim bandwidth, reset your nervous system, and remember you're human, not a productivity machine.

Mindfulness is neurological, not mystical. It strengthens the brain, regulates the nervous system, and restores your capacity to respond instead of react. You don't need a monastery or a Himalayan salt lamp. You just need a pause. Every breath is an invitation back to yourself.

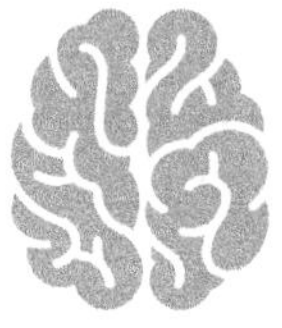

**CHAPTER 17.5**

# TL;DR, DO THIS NOW, AND CLINICAL CUES

## ☑ TL;DR

- Mindfulness is neuroscience in action. You're training your brain, not surrendering it.
- Mindfulness means noticing, not clearing. One breath, one pause, one unclenched jaw. That's enough.
- Your nervous system loves this. Every mindful pause signals safety, calming your amygdala and strengthening your vagal tone.
- Micromoments count. Try three breaths at a stoplight, noticing your coffee before sipping, or putting your phone down for sixty seconds.
- Skeptic-friendly entry point: dishes, showers, dog walks. Everyday life is already your meditation mat.

## ☑ Do This Now

Stop reading for thirty seconds. Breathe in. Breathe out. Notice your shoulders. That's mindfulness, and your brain just got a tiny workout.

## ☑ Clinical Cues

### ▨ Telomere Length (specialty lab)

- Optimal range/target: Healthy adults typically show 5,000 to 15,000 base pairs in leukocyte telomere length. What matters most is the rate of shortening over time; slowing or stabilizing telomere loss is the gold-standard indicator of healthier aging.

**Why it matters:** Chronic stress accelerates telomere erosion, which is linked to earlier cellular aging, inflammation, and higher risk of chronic disease. Mindfulness, stress reduction, and aerobic movement have repeatedly been shown to slow telomere shortening, essentially helping the body age more slowly.

### ▨ Epigenetic Aging Clocks (DNA methylation panels)

- Optimal range/target: Your biological age ideally matches or trails your birthday age by zero to three years. A biological age that is two to three-plus years older than your chronological age is a clinical red flag for stress dysregulation, chronic inflammation, metabolic strain, and accelerated disease risk.

**Why it matters:** DNA methylation is one of the strongest biomarkers of stress load. When your biology is aging faster than your calendar age, it signals that your stress system is burning too hot. Mindfulness practices, sleep consistency, healthy relationships, and nervous system regulation have been shown to recalibrate methylation patterns toward lower biological age.

### ■ GABA (serum)

- Optimal range/target: adult serum reference ranges commonly fall around 0.02–0.07 μg/mL (20–70 ng/mL).
- Consistently below ~0.02 μg/mL is associated with anxiety, rumination, irritability, PMS symptoms, poor sleep quality, and difficulty settling the nervous system.

**Why it matters:** GABA is your brain's natural inhibitory chemical. It relaxes an overstimulated stress response, quiets racing thoughts, and helps the nervous system reenter parasympathetic mode. Low GABA means the brain struggles to shut off hypervigilance; mindfulness practices reliably raise GABA levels, supporting calm, focus, and emotional steadiness.

### Salivary Immunoglobulin A (sIgA)

- Optimal range/target: Typical healthy resting range sits around 100–600 µg/mL.
- Levels below ~100 µg/mL are linked to chronic stress load, higher viral susceptibility, slower healing, gastrointestinal vulnerability, and overall immune suppression.

**Why it matters:** sIgA is your frontline immune defense in saliva, gut, and mucosal tissues. Stress reliably suppresses sIgA, leaving you more vulnerable to infections and inflammatory cascades. Mindfulness and nervous system regulation have been shown to restore sIgA levels, improving immune protection and resilience under strain.

### EEG Neurofeedback Metrics (theta-to-beta ratio, alpha patterns)

- Optimal pattern targets:
  - Higher alpha (8–12 Hz): relaxation, creativity, emotional flexibility
  - Lower high beta (19–30 Hz): hyperarousal, anxiety, overthinking

In anxious brains, we typically see excess high beta and low alpha. A healthy, regulated profile shifts the ratio toward alpha dominance.

**Why it matters:** An anxious nervous system lives in high beta: scanning, predicting danger, and burning cognitive fuel. Mindfulness, breathwork, and meditation increase alpha rhythms and normalize beta activity. The shift reflects a brain that is calmer, less reactive, more socially open, and better able to recover after stress.

## ☑ Moving On

If mindfulness feels like magic, that's because your brain is literally rewiring itself every time you pause. And the scans prove it. In fact, the next chapter is where we get nerdy with MRIs, gray matter, and your very own "inner CEO" in the prefrontal cortex.

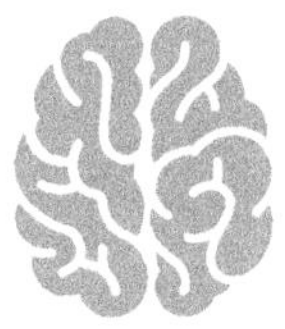



# CHAPTER 18

# YOUR BRAIN ON MINDFULNESS: THE NEUROSCIENCE OF PAYING ATTENTION

If you've ever wondered whether sitting still and breathing could actually do anything for your mental health, brace yourself: It can. We're talking structural, measurable, MRI scan–level changes in your brain. Mindfulness rewires your brain to be calmer all the time, beyond momentary calm. Let's get cozy with a few key brain regions and understand why mindfulness is basically a neurological power move.

## Gray Matter (And Why It Matters)

Your brain is made up of two main types of tissue: gray matter and white matter.

- Gray matter is the heavy lifter. It contains most of the brain's neuronal cell bodies and is involved in muscle control, decision-making, emotional regulation, memory, and yes, mindfulness. Think of it as your brain's headquarters.
- White matter is the communication highway. It's made of myelinated axons (nerve fibers wrapped in a fatty insulation layer) that let different brain regions talk to each other quickly and efficiently. Without it, your thoughts would crawl instead of connect.

The takeaway: Both matter, pun intended, but mindfulness has been shown to support healthier gray matter volume and function. More efficient headquarters. Better emotional regulation. Stronger cognitive control.

## The Prefrontal Cortex: Your Inner CEO

Sitting right behind your forehead, the prefrontal cortex is your brain's executive command center. It helps you plan, focus, regulate emotions, resist impulses, and basically act like a responsible adult.

It's the voice in your head that says, "Maybe don't send that angry email" or "We've had enough wine for a Tuesday."

**Key study:** A Harvard study in 2011 [Hölzel et al.] showed that just eight weeks of mindfulness meditation increased gray matter density in the prefrontal cortex. Translation: mindfulness literally bulked up the brain area responsible for wise decision-making, emotional balance, and self-control.

And here's the bigger picture: these changes aren't random. They're part of neuroplasticity, your brain's built-in ability to rewire itself through repeated experiences. Every time you pause to breathe instead of spiraling, you're training your neural circuits like a muscle. Over time, calm replaces panic as your default setting.

## The Amygdala: Your Inner Alarmist in Chief

Now, meet the fiery amygdala, your brain's alarm system. This almond-shaped cluster detects threats and flips the fight-or-flight switch. That's useful when you're crossing a busy street. Less useful when it's lighting up because your boss sends "Quick sync?" in an email with no context.

Chronic stress and trauma can make the amygdala hypersensitive, like a smoke alarm that shrieks every time you burn your toast.

Here's the good news: Mindfulness turns the volume down. That same Harvard study found decreased gray matter density in the amygdala after consistent meditation. Even better, the degree of shrinkage tracked directly with participants' self-reported stress reduction.

In plain English: Their brains stopped overreacting, and so did they.

> ## Case Study: Using Mindfulness to Train the Brain
>
> Jenna, a teacher and mom of two, lived with background anxiety that never switched off. She joined a local mindfulness course and started meditating for ten minutes a day. Within weeks, she noticed she didn't lose her cool when her kids refused shoes or when lesson plans derailed. She still had stress, but it didn't own her anymore.
>
> And Jenna's not alone. College students who practice mindfulness before exams perform better because their brains literally process stress differently. People with insomnia often use body scans, slowly relaxing each muscle to finally sleep through the night.
>
> Mindfulness isn't one-size-fits-all; it's versatile brain training.

## Mindfulness as Resilience Training

The practical impact? Resilience. Yes, mindfulness helps you chill in the moment but it also rewires your recovery system. You bounce back faster after conflict, calm down quicker after stress, and even support your immune system by lowering your cortisol and inflammation.

It's like upgrading your brain's shock absorbers: The bumps are still there, but you don't feel every jolt.

## Mindfulness and Cellular Immunity: Why Thoughts Speak Chemistry

When your brain believes you're under threat, your body doesn't fact-check. It flips the biochemical switches needed to survive catastrophe. Mindfulness interrupts those threat broadcasts at their root, and research shows it reduces the inflammatory chemical signals that chronic stress loves to amplify. Studies have measured lower IL-6, CRP, and TNF-$\alpha$ after consistent meditation practice, along with improvements in immune surveillance and faster resolution of inflammatory flare states. This is stress-signal withdrawal at the cellular level, not placebo or wishful thinking.

When your amygdala quiets and your prefrontal cortex takes command, your hypothalamic-pituitary-adrenal (HPA) axis follows suit. Cortisol peaks fall, autonomic balance stabilizes, and your metabolism stops acting like it's bracing for disaster. In that calmer terrain, your cellular energy production runs cleaner, damaging oxidative stress drops, and your brain's inflammatory chemistry shifts away from compounds that damage neurons. Markers of brain aging and cellular damage decline, while signals that promote brain growth and repair increase. Less inflammatory pressure equals more neurogenesis, clearer cognition, steadier mood, and a body that stops attacking itself just to survive another imaginary fire.

Mindfulness is biological diplomacy at the cellular level. It signals to your immune system that life is manageable, teaches responsiveness over reactivity, and interrupts the chronic stress patterns running your brain. When you change the way you relate to your thoughts, your cells hear it too.

## Mindfulness Is Basically Brain Botox

The benefits of mindfulness reach far beyond a calmer mood. They're visible in neuroimaging and clinical trials.

A large meta-analysis by Goyal and colleagues (2014), reviewing forty-seven randomized controlled trials, found that mindfulness meditation significantly reduced anxiety, depression, and psychological stress across diverse populations.

Another landmark neuroimaging study by Hölzel et al. (2011) showed that just eight weeks of mindfulness training increased hippocampal gray matter density (memory, learning, emotional regulation) and decreased amygdala density, correlating with reductions in perceived stress.

Translation: better focus, steadier mood, fewer internal alarms blaring.

Practicing mindfulness is like doing neural squats: Repetition reshapes the tissue itself. Each time you slow down, notice a thought, and return to the present moment, you're strengthening the networks responsible for emotional regulation, executive function, and perspective-taking while thinning the ones that catastrophize, overreact, or keep you in perpetual fight-or-flight mode.

That's the neuroscience behind the metaphor: Consistent reps build the structures you want and shrink the ones that make life harder. Mindfulness requires active training.

And you don't have to meditate for hours in a forest. Even five to ten minutes a day creates measurable shifts.

## A Note for Trauma Survivors

One important caveat: If you've experienced trauma—certain mindfulness practices; like closing your eyes and turning inward—can feel overwhelming. That doesn't mean mindfulness isn't for you. It just means you may need to start differently.

Grounding practices like mindful walking, focusing on external sounds, or holding a textured object can be safer starting points. Mindfulness adapts to you: sitting still, mindful walking, or grounding exercises (especially important if trauma makes closing your eyes feel unsafe).

Mindfulness thickens your prefrontal cortex, quiets your amygdala, supports your hippocampus, and rewires your stress response.

So the next time someone tells you mindfulness is "just breathing," you can smile and say, "Actually, it's science. My brain has receipts."

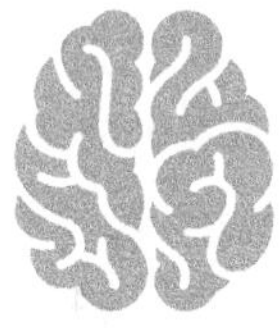



# TL;DR, DO THIS NOW, AND CLINICAL CUES

## ☑ TL;DR

- Mindfulness literally changes your brain: It bulks up your prefrontal cortex (focus, emotional regulation) and calms down your amygdala (fear, overreaction).
- Neuroplasticity means your brain is trainable. Every mindful pause is a rep in the gym of rewiring.
- Consistent practice builds resilience: faster recovery after stress, steadier emotions, even stronger immunity.
- It's not one-size-fits-all: Mindfulness can be sitting still, mindful walking, or grounding exercises (especially important if trauma makes closing your eyes feel unsafe).
- MRI scans don't lie: Five to ten minutes a day is enough to make measurable changes in brain structure and mood.

## ☑ **Do This Now**

1. Micropause practice: Take three slow breaths before opening your inbox, responding to a text, or walking into a meeting.
2. Body scan in bed: Notice each body part and let it soften; this is great for sleep or unwinding.
3. Mindful walk: Skip the podcast for once. Just notice your steps, your breath, and what's around you.
4. Grounding for anxious days: Name five things you see, four you hear, three you touch, two you smell, one you taste.
5. Start where you are: Don't aim for thirty minutes, aim for two. Build from there.

## ☑ **Clinical Cues**

### ▪ **Brain-Derived Neurotrophic Factor (BDNF)**

**Why it matters:** Mindfulness increases BDNF, the brain's "fertilizer" for neuroplasticity, synaptic growth, memory, and emotional resilience. Low BDNF has been linked to depression, cognitive decline, and poor stress recovery.

BDNF lacks a universally accepted population reference range; different assays vary widely. But clinicians typically look for values on the higher end of the laboratory's published range rather than the low-normal edge. Persistently low BDNF may warrant a conversation about chronic stress load, inflammation, sleep deprivation, or antidepressant response. [Zoladz, J.A., and Pilc, A. (2010). *Journal of Physiology and Pharmacology*]

## ▪ Neurofilament Light Chain (serum or CSF)

**Why it matters:** NfL is emerging as a marker of axonal injury, neurodegeneration, and brain aging. Mindfulness has been shown to lower NfL signaling, suggesting reduced inflammatory stress on neural tissue.

In healthy adults, NfL levels tend to remain low and stable. Significant increases over time, or values above the upper limit of the laboratory's reference range, can be a cue to investigate chronic inflammation, sleep apnea, long-term stress physiology, or traumatic brain injury history. [Khalil, M. et al. (2018). Neurofilaments as biomarkers in neurological disorders. *Nature Reviews Neurology,* 14, 577–589. https://doi.org/10.1038/s41582-018-0058-z]

## ▪ EEG and qEEG Biomarkers

**Why it matters:** Mindfulness strengthens frontal lobe regulation and increases alpha rhythms (associated with calm focus, creativity, emotional integration, and reduced distractibility). Women with ADHD-like symptoms or scattered attention often show measurable shifts here.

On EEG, clinicians tend to look for:

- Robust alpha activity (especially 8–12 Hz) during resting states
- Reduced excessive high-beta activity (associated with anxiety, overthinking, hypervigilance)

Patterns, not perfection, matter. Shift toward dominant alpha is often interpreted as improved executive functioning and emotional regulation. [Lomas, T. et al. (2015) *Neuroscience & Biobehavioral Reviews*]

## ▦ Alpha and Theta Power (neurofeedback panels)

**Why it matters:** High-quality research shows mindfulness increases alpha and theta power, correlating with relaxed focus, insight, creativity, and balanced arousal. It's the sweet spot between "switched on" and "scattered."

Practitioners often look for:

- Balanced alpha-to-theta ratio (not suppressed, not dominant)
- Increases in alpha waves over time during meditative practice
- Fewer spikes in high-beta and reactivity

The direction of change matters more than any fixed numeric target. [Ahani, A. et al. (2014)]

## ▦ Dopamine Metabolites (Organic Acids Test)

**Why it matters:** Dopamine metabolism reflects attention, motivation, reward sensitivity, and impulse control. Poor conversion or sluggish breakdown can mirror symptoms like low drive, anhedonia, impaired focus, or internal restlessness.

Rather than rigid cutoffs, clinicians evaluate:

- Whether dopamine metabolites sit comfortably within the middle-to-upper portion of the reference range
- Whether values are persistently low (low motivation, fatigue, distractibility) or persistently high (restlessness, irritability, impulsivity)

Stable, mid-range patterns suggest balanced signaling, while chronic extremes may be a cue to explore sleep, nutrient status, stress burden, ADHD traits, or antidepressant use. [Gao, J. et al. (2020).]

## ☑ Moving On

You now know that mindfulness reshapes the very structures of your brain, beyond making you feel calmer. It thickens your decision-making circuits, tones down your inner alarm system, and gives you tools to recover from stress faster. Even with all that, most of us are still walking around with a mental radio station playing in the background and not always the good kind.

That constant hum of self-talk, the daydream loops, the random flashbacks at 2 a.m.? That's your default mode network (DMN), and it's the playlist that decides how you feel about yourself when you're not even paying attention. In the next chapter, we'll meet your DMN, learn why it can be both your best friend and your worst critic, and, most importantly, figure out how to change the station when it won't shut up.

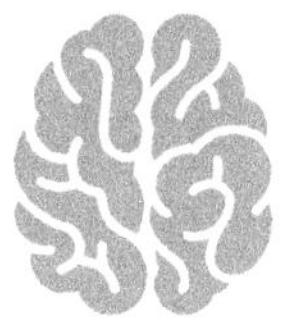



# CHAPTER 19

# THE DEFAULT MODE NETWORK: HOW TO CHANGE THE STATION IN YOUR HEAD

Let me tell you a story.

A few years ago, a woman I'll call Claire walked into her therapist's office looking . . . muted. Not sad. Not angry. Just like someone had dimmed the lights inside her. Claire used to be sharp, quick-witted, and that friend who could turn any bad day into a comedy sketch. Now? She was running on fumes. Every morning, she woke up to the same internal broadcast: "You're failing. You've always been failing."

That voice wasn't "the truth." It was her default mode network (DMN), the part of the brain that plays your personal highlight reel on repeat, whether or not it's accurate. And Claire's reel? It was a season-long binge of self-criticism and doomscrolls.

Her therapist explained two things that would change her life: the reticular activating system (RAS), her brain's filter for what she notices, and neuroplasticity, the fact that she could rewire her own mental broadcast. Over the next six months, they worked on tiny, deliberate habits: writing down one thing she wanted to notice each day, catching negative loops in the moment, and rehearsing new thoughts out loud. Slowly, her DMN stopped playing the "You're failing" show and switched to "You've survived worse, you can handle this." One day she said, "It's like my brain flipped the channel, and now I can finally hear myself again." That, my friend, is the miracle: Your brain is returnable.

## Meet Your DMN: The Brain's Background Radio Station

The default mode network, discovered in 2001 by neurologist Marcus Raichle, is a set of brain regions that light up when you're not focused on the outside world. It's the mental space where shower thoughts, random daydreams, and intrusive "remember that time" memories live. It's also the seat of your self-talk, the constant commentary about who you are and how you're doing.

The problem? The DMN plays whatever you've rehearsed most, helpful or not. If you've been rehearsing anxiety and criticism for years, that becomes the default playlist. If you've been practicing gratitude and agency, that's what it will play instead.

## The RAS–DMN Tag Team

This is where Mel Robbins's explanation clicks. In her conversation with neurosurgeon Dr. Jim Doty, she describes the reticular activating system (RAS) as the brain's "attention filter." It notices what you've told it matters and begins selecting information that matches that intention while ignoring the rest. Say "I'm looking for a new car," and you suddenly start spotting that exact model everywhere. Decide "I want to be more confident," and your RAS begins tagging examples that support confidence, not insecurity.

From there, the habit loops travel to the default mode network (DMN), the brain's internal narrator. The DMN stores the stories you repeat about yourself and your life, and it plays them on autopilot. The RAS decides what gets in; the DMN decides what meaning you attach to it. If your DMN script is "I always get this wrong," your RAS will happily pull evidence to confirm it. If you begin practicing a different internal story, "I figure things out," the RAS starts noticing proof, and the DMN updates to believe it.

This is how neuroplasticity works at the behavioral level.

## The Science of Change

Neuroplasticity is your brain's ability to change. It's one of the most well-documented facts in neuroscience. Here's a brief history:

- 1793: Michele Malacarne showed that animals trained in skills had bigger, more developed cerebellums than untrained ones.

- 1964: Marian Diamond proved that adult brains can grow and adapt with learning and stimulation.
- 1990s onward: Michael Merzenich demonstrated that even after injury, the brain can reorganize itself, and targeted mental exercises can rival medication in treating certain disorders.

Psychologist William James said it best more than a century ago: "The greatest discovery of my generation is that a human being can alter his life by altering his attitudes." Modern neuroscience would add: Altering our attitudes alters how our neurons fire together; and whatever fires together, wires together.

## Neuroplasticity: Why Your Brain Changes When You Practice

Your brain is a set of emotional habits, or a predetermined wiring map. It is elastic tissue that constantly remodels itself based on what you repeatedly pay attention to, what signals you send through it, and whether the biological environment is supportive enough to build new connections. This ability to rewire and reorganize is called neuroplasticity, and it's the core mechanism behind hope, recovery, learning, and emotional change.

Every thought pattern is a circuit.

Every coping style is a learned algorithm.

Every instinctive reaction—spiraling, catastrophizing, shutting down, perfectionism—is a neural pathway that your brain chose because it once solved a problem.

Neuroplasticity is how you teach it new options.

Here's the process in plain English:

1. **Repetition creates wiring.**
   The circuits you run the most become the easiest for your brain to default to. Rumination, vigilance, people-pleasing, intrusive loops, self-criticism: They strengthen through rehearsal. That's your brain being efficient.

2. **Attention directs change.**
   When you shift focus to grounding, reframing, sensory awareness, breathwork, or curiosity instead of self-attack, the brain literally reroutes electrical traffic and prunes old pathways to make new patterns easier to access.

3. **Biology determines the quality of rewiring.**
   Sleep consolidates new neural links. Omega-3s improve membrane fluidity. B vitamins support neurotransmitter synthesis. Iron delivers oxygen. Magnesium calms excitatory noise. Stable glucose prevents inflammatory interference. Your brain can't upgrade in starvation mode.

4. **Practice becomes structure.**
   Over weeks and months, the new patterns stop being something you "try." They become automatic preferences built into the architecture: calmer reflexes, more flexible thinking, emotional steadiness, and a lower threshold for joy.

This is why the strategies in this book aren't coping mechanisms. They're training signals. You're changing how your brain interprets stress, regulates emotion, and interacts with your life—retraining, not just managing.

So when you repeat something like grounding, breathwork, intentional thought selection, mindful movement, or cognitive reappraisal, don't underestimate it. You are running a neurochemical command that tells your brain to redesign itself.

And that's the most honest definition of healing: biological change through consistent signals.

## When You're Running on Empty

When you're in that energy-empty, not-quite-yourself phase where even making coffee feels like wading through molasses, your DMN is usually serving up the worst reruns in its archive. The good news? You can change the station.

Mindfulness meditation, journaling, reframing thoughts in therapy, gratitude practice—all of these interrupt old wiring and lay down new neural tracks. Do it often enough, and you train your DMN to default to something more useful than "You're failing at life."

Neuroscientist Susan Whitfield-Gabrieli's brain-imaging research shows that these shifts are visible on scans. After consistent mindfulness practice, people's DMNs begin activating in different patterns: Regions involved in rumination and self-criticism quiet down, while networks tied to emotional regulation, present-moment awareness, and perspective-taking strengthen. In plain English? The stories your brain loops, the tone of your inner narration, and the meaning you assign to your experiences become measurably calmer, clearer, and less catastrophic.

## The Payoff of a Rewired DMN

When you change your default thought patterns, you're restructuring the physical pathways that run your mental life. The results are concrete:

- Less mental noise and fewer negative spirals
- Sharper focus and better decision-making
- More energy and motivation
- A grounded, steady sense of yourself, even in chaos

You can't stop your brain from running its background station, but you *can* choose the playlist. And once you learn how, you'll wonder why you ever let the old station run the show.

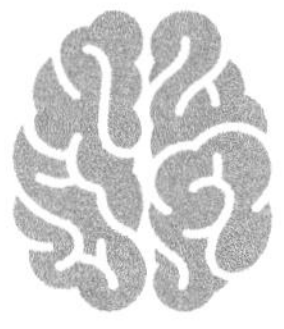



# TL;DR, DO THIS NOW, AND CLINICAL CUES

## ☑ TL;DR

- Your default mode network (DMN) is your brain's background station, looping whatever self-narrative you've rehearsed most, good or bad.

- The reticular activating system (RAS) is your attention filter; it shows you proof of whatever you've told your brain matters.

- Together, the RAS feeds your DMN, and your DMN interprets what it means about you.

- Neuroplasticity means you can rewire both. Fire new thoughts often enough, and they become your brain's new default.

- When you're in an energy-empty, off-your-game phase, shifting your default script changes not just your mindset, but your brain itself.

## ☑ Do This Now

Reboot your DMN:

1. Name your current loop.
   - Spend a day noticing the most common thought your brain serves up about *you*. ("I'm behind," "I can't keep up," etc.) Write it down. Yes, on paper.
2. Choose your upgrade script.
   - Replace it with a believable, useful alternative. ("I figure things out." "I'm learning faster than I think.") Avoid toxic positivity; you're going for *credible*, not *Pinterest*.
3. Prime your RAS.
   - Each morning, tell your brain what to look for that day. Example: "Show me proof I'm resourceful." Your RAS will scan your environment to match that instruction.
4. Interrupt and swap.
   - When you catch the old loop, literally say "switch" (out loud or in your head) and drop in the new one.
5. Rehearse daily.
   - Write, say, or visualize your upgrade script at least three times a day. Repetition = rewiring.
   - Pro tip: Pair this with something you already do every day like brushing your teeth or making coffee so your DMN upgrade becomes as automatic as your caffeine habit.

## ☑ Clinical Cues

### ▣ Kynurenine-to-Tryptophan Ratio

- Optimal: <0.04 (4%)

**Why it matters:** When inflammation is low, less tryptophan gets siphoned into the kynurenine pathway and more is available to make serotonin. Higher ratios correlate with neuroinflammation, anxious rumination, irritability, and depressive looping. Lower ratios tend to predict calmer mood, better cognitive flexibility, and fewer "sticky" thoughts.

### ▣ Glutamate-to-GABA Balance

- Optimal glutamate <20 μmol/L, GABA 700–1200 nmol/L

**Why it matters:** Glutamate fuels alarm states and mental noise; GABA is the brake pedal. A healthy brain keeps glutamate modest and GABA strong enough to buffer stress. When glutamate runs high and GABA is low, the DMN becomes overactive, producing insomnia spirals, catastrophic thinking, and looping inner narratives.

### ▣ Phosphatidylserine and Choline

- Optimal phosphatidylserine 60–100 μg/mL; Choline 7–10 μmol/L

**Why it matters:** These nutrients maintain neuronal membranes, stabilize electrical signaling, and support clear thinking. Low levels often show up in people with emotional reactivity, brain fog, menopausal cognitive shifts, and difficulty regulating attention. When they're restored to optimal, DMN firing becomes more efficient and less erratic.

## Quinolinic Acid

- Optimal: <0.80 ng/mL

**Why it matters:** Quinolinic acid is an inflammatory metabolite that overstimulates NMDA receptors and acts like jet fuel on DMN hyperactivity. People with elevated levels frequently describe relentless worry loops, obsessive analysis, and difficulty turning down their inner narrator. Bringing this marker down usually parallels quieter self-talk and more emotional ease.

## EEG/fMRI Signatures

There's no single "lab value," but a well-regulated DMN shows less hyperactivity in the medial prefrontal cortex and stronger connection with executive control networks. On EEG, that usually looks like calmer alpha dominance at rest and balanced theta-to-beta rhythms. These patterns are considered the gold-standard evidence that the brain's storytelling system is actually rewiring. In trials, these signatures consistently predict reduced rumination and better mood regulation.

## ☑ **Moving On**

Now you know mindfulness is literal brain renovation, shrinking your amygdala, thickening your prefrontal cortex, and teaching your default mode network to calm the hell down. Knowing the science doesn't change your life. Doing it does. Most people trip up because life is loud, time is scarce, and nobody wants one more thing to fail at. The good news? You don't need a monastery, a yoga mat, or a single stick of incense. You just need a few practical, real-world ways to slip mindfulness into the chaos you're already living. Which brings us to your next chapter: the zero-guilt menu of practices you can start today, even if your brain currently feels like a phone that's been at 1% battery for the last three years.

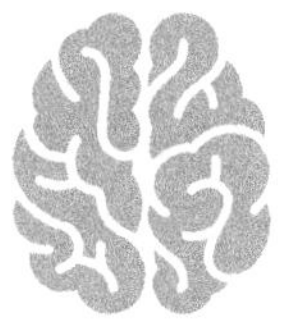



# PRACTICE MAKES PEACE: EVERYDAY MINDFULNESS FOR THE BUSY, BURNED-OUT, OR SKEPTICAL

Have you noticed the people who need mindfulness the most are the ones least likely to believe they have time for it? If you've ever said, "I can't meditate; I have things to do," congratulations: You're exactly who this section is for.

Because somewhere between the mental to-do list that never ends and the lunch you ate while standing at the counter, there is space. Not a spa day. Not a silent retreat. Just . . . space. Room to breathe. And more importantly, room to think clearly and feel less like you're living on the edge of a nervous breakdown.

Mindfulness is about noticing when you're about to crash and giving yourself an off-ramp. And that skill? It's trainable. You don't have to light a candle, sit cross-legged, or download yet another app you won't open. You just have to practice.

Practice makes peace. But only if you actually do it.

## 1. Mindful Breathing (One-to-Two Minutes That Can Save Your Whole Day)

*What it is:*

This is the "entry-level" mindfulness move, but don't underestimate it. Just one to two minutes of focusing on your breath can flip your brain from full-blown panic to functional adult. No incense, no chanting. Just you and your lungs.

*How to do it:*

- Inhale slowly for four seconds.
- Exhale slowly for six.
- Repeat for one to two minutes.

*What's actually happening:*

You're activating your parasympathetic nervous system (a.k.a. your "rest and digest" mode), which slows your heart rate and tells your brain you're safe. Science even shows that microdoses of mindfulness, just sixty seconds, can measurably reduce anxiety and improve focus. [Zeidan et al. (2010)]

*When to use it:*

Before a meeting. After a tense conversation. Mid-scroll when your brain starts catastrophizing. Or literally whenever you remember you have lungs.

## 2. The STOP Method (When Life Is Giving Full-Crisis Energy)

STOP is an acronym that gives your overwhelmed brain a sequence it can follow. It's like mindfulness with a cheat sheet.

- S: Stop what you're doing.
- T: Take a breath. Seriously. Just one will do.
- O: Observe what's happening. (What am I feeling? What's going on around me?)
- P: Proceed with intention. (Now what? How do I want to respond?)

Aim for awareness, not perfection. Imagine applying this in the middle of a stress spiral instead of unleashing a rage text or inhaling a family-sized bag of tortilla chips. Now *that's* nervous system power.

*Micro Story:* One of my clients started using STOP before opening her inbox. Within two weeks, she said mornings went from "panic storm" to "low-key drizzly rain." Still annoying, but manageable.

## 3. Single-Tasking + Sensory Awareness (The Most Mindful Thing You're Not Doing)

Multitasking is a myth. You're doing five things poorly while stressing about a sixth.

Pick one daily activity and turn it into a sensory check-in:

- Washing your hands: Feel the water. Smell the soap. Listen to the sound. Boom, mindful moment.
- Drinking coffee: Stop gulping. Actually taste it. Pretend you're auditioning for a Folgers commercial.
- Showering: Feel the temperature. Hear the water. Bonus: Since you're already naked, try a body scan too.

Mindfulness can be as simple as doing what you already do but consciously.

## 4. Mindful Walking (No Robes. No Gongs. Just You + Feet.)

You need your body in motion. No foggy mountain or Zen master required.

*How to do it:*

- Put your phone away (really).
- Walk at a natural pace.
- Notice your steps, your arms swinging, the sounds around you.

- When your mind wanders (and it will), gently bring it back to your feet.

Walking this way turns a commute or errand into a nervous system reset. Science backs this up: Research shows that mindful walking activates the parasympathetic branch of the autonomic nervous system, which supports digestion, lowers perceived stress, and even enhances cognitive flexibility and creative thinking. [Gotink et al. (2015); Russell et al. (2019); Oppezzo and Schwartz (2014)] Basically, it's multitasking for your *nervous system* instead of your inbox.

## 5. Three-Minute Body Scan (For Bedtime or Anytime You Need to Unclench)

Perfect for those of us who carry stress like it's our emotional purse.

*How to do it:*

- Lie down and close your eyes.
- Start at your toes and move up: feet, legs, hips, chest, arms, face.
- Just notice sensations. No judgment, no fixing.

It's like tucking your nervous system into bed. Great for nights when your brain wants to replay every embarrassing moment since 2007.

## Making It Stick (Without Feeling Like You're Failing)

Here's the part most people miss: the practice only matters if it's doable.

- Start pathetically small. One breath. One minute. That's enough. Consistency beats intensity.
- Attach it to something you already do. Breathe while the coffee brews. Scan your body after brushing your teeth.
- Let it be imperfect. You'll get distracted, forget, or feel silly. That *is* the practice. Every time you notice and come back? That's a rep.
- Track how you feel, not how long. Ask "Did I feel even 5% calmer?" If yes, you won.

## Mindfulness for Skeptics

Mindfulness is not:

- A cult
- A productivity hack in disguise
- Spiritual bypassing where you pretend problems don't exist

Mindfulness is:

- Nervous system training
- Emotional regulation you can practice anywhere
- Presence, not perfection

## Bonus: Mindful Living Across the Board

Mindfulness isn't just for sitting still. It makes workouts feel stronger (because you notice your body), meals more satisfying (because you actually taste them), and conversations deeper (because you're actually listening).

If you want to take it further:

- Try an MBSR (mindfulness-based stress reduction) course.
- Experiment with evidence-based apps (Headspace, Healthy Minds, Ten Percent Happier).
- Add journal prompts: "What did I notice today? When did I feel safe? When did I feel triggered?"

You spend so much of your life knowing other people: what they need, what they expect, how they feel. But you? You deserve to know yourself: your patterns, your triggers, your breakthroughs. Mindfulness is about meeting yourself in real time and remembering this: Peace is a trainable skill, not a gift. It's a skill. And you're allowed to learn it.

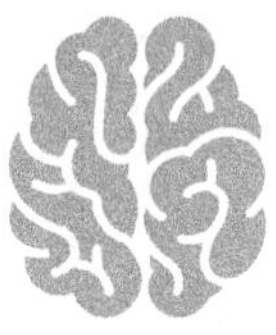

**CHAPTER 20.5**

# TL;DR, DO THIS NOW, AND CLINICAL CUES

## ☑ TL;DR

- Forget incense and retreats; mindfulness is about catching spirals before they own you.
- Even microdoses (sixty seconds!) can calm your nervous system and retrain your brain.
- Five simple practices work anywhere: mindful breathing, STOP method, single-tasking with sensory awareness, mindful walking, and body scans.
- Consistency > intensity. One breath daily is better than a thirty-minute meditation you never do.
- Mindfulness means practice, not perfection. Getting distracted and returning? That's the win.

## ☑ Do This Now

- Pick one practice and attach it to something you already do (e.g., one mindful breath while coffee brews).
- Use STOP before your next stress trigger: inbox, traffic, or tough convo.
- Try a mindful walk today, even for five minutes, without your phone.
- Tonight: Perform a three-minute body scan before bed instead of doomscrolling.
- Journal prompt: "What did I notice about myself today that I normally miss?"

## ☑ Clinical Cues

### ▣ Salivary Immunoglobulin A (sIgA)

- Optimal range: >100–300 µg/mL (Ranges vary by lab.)

**Why it matters:** Even five to ten minutes of mindfulness can raise sIgA, your first-line immune defense. Low sIgA is common in chronically stressed women. It shows up as frequent colds, gut irritation, and immune fatigue.

### ▣ Telomere Length (specialty test)

- Optimal target: telomere length at or above the expected range for age

**Why it matters:** Daily micropractices of mindfulness reduce inflammatory signaling that accelerates telomere shortening. Translation: Short mindful pauses literally slow cellular aging. Women in their thirties to fifties often test "older" biologically; mindfulness helps reverse that drift.

### Epigenetic Methylation Age (DNA methylation panels)

- Optimal target: biological age at or below chronological age

**Why it matters:** Consistent mindfulness downregulates pro-inflammatory genes, improves methylation patterns, and keeps your biological age lower than your driver's license says. These practices change your code and genetic expression, not just emotional state.

### Alpha-Amylase (salivary stress marker)

- Optimal range: <60–70 U/mL at rest (Ranges depends on collection timing.)

**Why it matters:** Alpha-amylase drops quickly after even short mindfulness sessions. For women skeptical of meditation, this marker often feels validating: It shows the nervous system literally shifting out of fight-or-flight mode within minutes.

### ▨ GABA (serum)

- Optimal range: 0.30–1.50 mg/L (Ranges vary by assay.)

**Why it matters:** Mindfulness boosts GABA, which quiets the anxious, overactive mind. The increase is measurable and often clinically meaningful in women with insomnia, racing thoughts, and PMS irritability.

Your nervous system doesn't need grand gestures. It needs reps. One mindful moment at a time builds a calmer, more resilient you.

## ☑ Moving On

You now have a tool kit of practices that prove mindfulness is practical nervous system training. And there's more to build on. The roots of mindfulness stretch back through Buddhist philosophy and other ancient schools that understood the same core truth: Resilience begins in the mind and body.

Before we move forward, here's a bridge you'll need.

The ancients focused on breath work to teach something deeper: how to respond to the world instead of reacting to it. That's where we pivot into a companion philosophy that quietly shaped Western psychological thinking long before therapy was a field at all: Stoicism.

The Stoics were the original calm-in-chaos thinkers. Long before meditation apps, they taught the same fundamentals you've been practicing: Notice what's yours to control, drop what isn't, and stay present instead of spiraling.

So if mindfulness teaches us how to pause and pay attention, Stoicism teaches us what to do with the space that pause creates. One strengthens the nervous system; the other strengthens the response. Together, they form a natural pairing, two different lenses pointed at the same goal: a steadier inner climate, no matter the weather.

And that's where we're headed next.

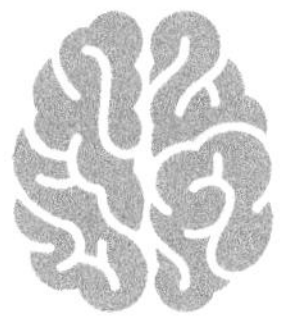



# CHAPTER 21

# CONTROL FREAKS, MEET THE STOICS

Marcus Aurelius called, and he said, "Chill."

Before mindfulness apps, guided meditations, and therapists with calming voices and throw pillows, there were Stoics. They were Roman emperors, philosophers, exiled statesmen, and former slaves who learned how to keep their minds intact while the world around them was fully unhinged. If you've ever tried to stay calm in traffic, survive a group chat meltdown, or not snowball over a text that just reads "k," you've already started dabbling in Stoicism. Welcome to the club. Togas optional.

## Control What You Can. Leave the Rest. Seriously.

At the heart of Stoic philosophy is one truth that's both liberating and annoying in its simplicity: Some things are within your control, and some things aren't. That's it. That's the tweet. The rest of Stoicism is essentially helping you emotionally survive this fact.

You can control your thoughts, your actions, your choices, your attitude, and on a good day, your breath. You can't control your ex, your boss's mood swings, your friend's passive-aggressive Instagram captions, or global inflation. Yet we ruminate, obsess, and doomscroll like our worry will help us.

Every time we try to mentally manhandle something that isn't ours to control—whether it's someone else's behavior, a missed opportunity, or the past—we drain energy we could be using to move forward. The Stoics got this. Epictetus, a Stoic philosopher who started life as a slave, put it bluntly: "Make the best use of what is in your power, and take the rest as it happens."

Modern research on cognitive reappraisal and reframing how we interpret a situation shows it *literally calms the nervous system.* Brain imaging studies reveal that reappraisal reduces activation in the amygdala (your fear center) and boosts regulation from the prefrontal cortex (your inner CEO). [Ochsner and Gross (2005)] This is stress relief written in neurons, not just philosophy.

## Accept What You Can't (Without the Meltdown)

Stoicism means practicing radical acceptance, not to give up, but to stop resisting reality.

This part is hard, especially if you're a type A, hyper-capable human who's used to muscling your way through life. Accepting what you can't control is wise, not weak. Protective, not passive. It keeps your mental energy from getting hijacked by things that are, quite frankly, not your circus and not your monkeys.

Acceptance ≠ approval. You can accept that someone hurt you without saying it was okay. You can accept that something happened without loving it. Acceptance is simply the pause between "This sucks" and "Okay, now what?"

## Don't Let Your Emotions Drive the Chariot (They Can Ride in the Back Seat)

Imagine your mind as a chariot. Logic is holding the reins, steering you down the path. Then there are your emotions: fiery, passionate, dramatic, all trying to grab the wheel and screaming, "Let's drive straight into this field of panic and regret!"

Stoicism teaches you to let emotions ride along, but not to let them steer. Stoics felt deeply, but they practiced regulation over reactivity. Feel your feelings? Absolutely. Be ruled by them? Hard pass.

Your peace isn't up for group approval. It lives in your actions, not their opinions.

Neuroscience agrees: When we practice observing emotions instead of fusing with them, the prefrontal cortex strengthens, and the stress response chills out. That's regulation, not repression.

## Marcus Aurelius, Your Ancient Mental Health Coach

Ah! Marcus, the Stoic icon, part philosopher, part emperor, part burnt-out middle manager of the Roman Empire. Even Marcus Aurelius was drowning in imperial tasks written on wax tablets and papyrus. The medium changes; the stress response doesn't. He ruled during wars, plagues, and political chaos. Yet his private journal, written for no one but himself, became a manual for emotional resilience.

In *Meditations,* he wrote, "If you are distressed by anything external, the pain is not due to the thing itself, but to your estimate of it; and this you have the power to revoke at any moment."

Translation: That email, comment, or side-eye? The story you tell about it matters more than the event itself. But guess what? You can edit the story.

Another classic from Marcus: "If it's endurable, then endure it." A bit Spartan to modern ears, but the heart of it tracks with what we know about cognitive load. The more we stew in resistance and complaint, the less bandwidth we have left for clarity, problem-solving, and emotional regulation. Stoicism isn't about stuffing feelings or pretending nothing hurts. It's about clearing the mental fog so you can respond rather than react. Marcus didn't preach serenity from a spa; he found stillness in battle tents because he understood the upside: When you stop wrestling the moment, you get energy back to shape the next one. Stoicism is about clarity, presence, and perspective. He was practicing a kind of mindfulness long before it was branded and turned into an app.

## Stoicism + Mindfulness = Mental Health Power Couple

The overlap between Stoicism and mindfulness is uncanny. Both train you to notice your thoughts instead of automatically believing them. Both teach you to stay with the present moment rather than overanalyzing into prediction or regret. And both ask you to detach from drama, including your own, so you can respond from clarity instead of panic.

In fact, Stoic thought is the skeleton under modern cognitive behavioral therapy. Approaches like cognitive behavioral therapy (CBT) and acceptance and commitment therapy (ACT) borrow directly from Stoic principles: Observe, don't attach, redirect attention, and question the story your brain is telling you.

Where mindfulness asks, "What am I experiencing right now?" Stoicism follows with, "Is this interpretation accurate, helpful, or necessary?" One regulates the nervous system; the other interrogates the narrative.

Together, they make everyday life less reactive and more intentional. And you don't need a monastery or a toga to blend them. Try these simple combinations:

- Notice a wave of anxiety in your body. Mindfulness step: Name it without judgment. Stoic step: Ask whether the thought behind it is factual or just anticipatory wiring.
- When you catch your brain forecasting disaster, pause. Mindfulness step: Breathe into the present moment. Stoic step: Evaluate what's actually in your control, and act only on that.

- When someone irritates you, mindfulness gives you space before you respond. Stoicism helps you choose the response that aligns with your values rather than your reflex.

This synergy matters because it frees up executive function. When you stop fusing with every storyline your brain produces, you reclaim cognitive energy for perspective, planning, and behavior change. Call it what it is: trained attention plus trained interpretation.

## In Real Life, Detachment ≠ Disconnection

Stoic detachment means caring without drowning. When you're not tangled in your own emotional static, your brain has more bandwidth to read situations accurately. You stop mistaking impulse for insight. You stop outsourcing your peace to other people's behavior. You still feel, grieve, love, and show up. But you do it from a steadier nervous system and a clearer mind.

It's the difference between being inside a storm and watching one from a safe lookout. When you're soaked and scrambling, you can barely think about anyone but yourself. When you're dry and grounded, you can actually understand what the people in the rain might need and respond with something useful, not reactive.

## The Bridge Eastward: Head Meets Heart

We've seen how Stoicism sharpens the head. It challenges distorted thoughts, asks for clarity before emotion, and trains the mind to sort what you can influence from what you can't. The result is psychological steadiness instead of reflex. Cognitive mastery needs a partner. Once the noise quiets, how do you meet your inner world with compassion?

This is where Buddhism and mindfulness walk into the frame. While Stoicism strengthens discernment, Eastern practice strengthens compassion. Where the Stoic asks, "Is this story accurate or useful?" mindfulness asks, "Can I sit with this moment as it is without flinching?" One provides the scalpel; the other, the soft hands that hold the incision site.

Modern neuroscience practically begs us to marry the two. Stoicism activates the prefrontal cortex, helping with cognitive reframing, emotional regulation, and inhibitory control. Mindfulness calms limbic activation and lowers inflammatory stress signaling. One regulates interpretation. The other regulates reactivity. Together, they produce psychological range: clarity without harshness, awareness without self-attack, stillness that doesn't numb you, and concern that isn't fused with panic.

Philosophically, the two line up as well. Stoics believed we suffer more in imagination than reality. Buddhists believed suffering blooms most intensely when we cling to what we want events to be rather than what they are. Both saw rumination as a thief. Both insisted that presence is power. Both held that emotional steadiness is not detachment from humanity but the precondition for empathy.

That's the deeper point. The fusion offers a neurological solution to the very modern problem of overthinking, self-pressure, and disconnection from the present. Stoicism trims the mental static. Mindfulness teaches you to greet what remains with warmth instead of self-surveillance. When the head and the heart cooperate, you care more cleanly, choose more deliberately, and relate to yourself with less resistance.

The combination is quiet confidence. Rational calm with emotional depth. The kind of inner alignment that makes life feel less like a problem to solve and more like something you can inhabit.

In a world that nudges the brain into panic loops, distraction, and constant external comparison, that union matters. Thought and presence. Clarity and compassion. Head and heart. East and West. This is the nervous system's true glow-up.

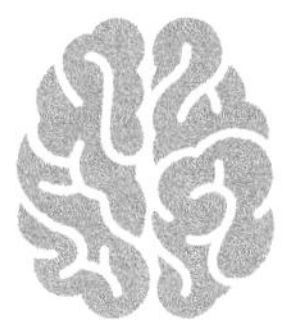



# TL;DR, DO THIS NOW, AND CLINICAL CUES

## ☑ TL;DR

- Stoicism = focusing on what's in your control, letting go of what isn't.
- Acceptance is not approval. It's pausing between "This sucks" and "Now what?"
- Emotions are passengers, not drivers. They can ride in the chariot, but they don't get the reins.
- Marcus Aurelius was basically journaling CBT centuries before it was trendy.
- Stoicism + mindfulness = head + heart. Logic + compassion. Rational calm + emotional presence.

## ☑ Do This Now

1. Ask the Stoic question. Next time you're in a ruminative thought loop, pause and ask, "Is this mine to control?" If yes, take a step. If no, release it.
2. Daily reframe: Catch one negative thought and rewrite it like Marcus would. Example: "This meeting will be a disaster" → "The meeting is outside my control. I can only prepare myself."
3. Practice Stoic journaling: Before bed, write down one thing that challenged you today and one way you handled it (or want to handle it better tomorrow).
4. Micromindfulness add-on: Pair the Stoic filter with a mindful breath. Inhale, exhale, *choose your focus.*
5. Boundary reminder: Caring wisely = emotional regulation. Choose where you spend your energy.

## ☑ Clinical Cues

Receipts that inner work shows up in lab data:

### Cortisol Awakening Response (CAR)

- Normal: 50–70% rise within thirty-to-forty-five minutes of waking
- Optimal: clean morning spike followed by gradual taper

**Why it matters:** If your mornings feel like wading through cement, check your CAR. Chronic stress or constant internal drama can flatten it, leaving you foggy, unmotivated, and dragging yourself through the day. Stoic-style mental discipline tamps down limbic overactivation and restores a healthy rise. Less catastrophic thinking → calmer threat response → stronger CAR. Motivation and clarity on tap, not borrowed from caffeine.

## ▪ Adrenaline and Noradrenaline (urinary catecholamines)

**Why it matters:** High catecholamines are basically your biochemistry screaming, "I'm on alert!" When your brain is busy predicting disaster, your adrenal system never stands down. Stoic practices train you to stop treating every discomfort like an emergency. That shift dials down false-alarm signaling and lowers catecholamine output. Translation: fewer irritable snap-reactions, less emotional edge, and more space in your head to actually think.

## ▪ Heart Rate Variability (HRV)

- Optimal: Higher is better.

**Why it matters:** HRV tanks when you're tight, hypercontrolling, and running on sympathetic fuel. Stoicism teaches one of the oldest nervous system hacks on record: Focus on what's within your control, and release what isn't. That cognitive reanchoring loosens the stress grip and nudges your autonomic system back toward balance. Higher HRV is the body saying, "I can flex, recover, and adapt." It's resilience in numbers.

### Salivary Alpha-Amylase (sAA)

**Why it matters:** sAA shoots up when your system is stuck in overdrive. It's the biochemical residue of white-knuckling your day. When you challenge catastrophic interpretations, stop personalizing everything, and abandon the idea that you have to micromanage the universe to feel safe, sAA goes down. That's not placebo; it's physiology. Mental steadiness shows up in your saliva.

### Kynurenine-to-Tryptophan Ratio

**Why it matters:** Stress reroutes tryptophan away from serotonin and into the inflammatory kynurenine pathway. That shift predicts low mood, irritability, brain fog, and existential dread spirals that feel inevitable. Stoic reframing and mindfulness practices cool the inflammatory response and redirect tryptophan back toward neurotransmitter balance. More serotonin available, less runaway rumination. Your calm has chemistry behind it.

## Moving On

So here we are, standing on the shoulders of Roman emperors and ancient philosophers, trying to navigate our own daily chaos with a bit more grace (and fewer mental meltdowns). Stoicism teaches us clarity and control. And it works best when combined with mindfulness and the Buddhist philosophy that produced it. One tradition sharpened the *head* with logic and perspective; the other softened the *heart* with compassion and awareness.

Millennia later, we get the best of both worlds: Stoic clarity + Buddhist mindfulness. Together, they create a blueprint for resilience that's more powerful than either on its own.

Which brings us to the next chapter: how Buddhist wisdom went from temple floors to therapy rooms and why this East-meets-West remix might just be the nervous system upgrade you've been waiting for.

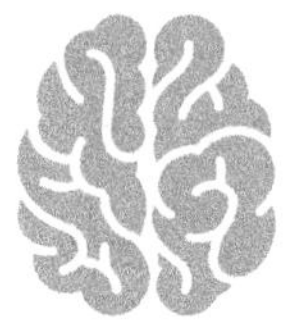



# CHAPTER 22

# OLD WISDOM, NEW ENERGY

The original mindfulness trailblazers were practicing presence long before it got rebranded as pseudo help in corporate wellness emails. Millennia before influencers started hashtagging their morning routines, Buddhist wisdom already had it nailed: Our minds love to overthink, replay, and catastrophize like it's their full-time job with no overtime pay. Their answer? Suffering and how to end it.

The liberation part comes next; stay with me.

## Buddhism Was Doing This Before It Was Cool

Buddhism doesn't just drop "good vibes only" platitudes. It lays out the human condition with brutal honesty. The Four Noble Truths are basically the OG self-help manual:

1. Life involves suffering (because, well, have you been alive lately?).
2. Suffering has a cause (craving, clinging, wishing things were different while still doomscrolling).
3. There's a way to stop suffering (cue the hope).
4. That way is the Eightfold Path (your guide to living with less chaos).

So, what does this actually look like in real life? It's taking awareness, ethics, and mental discipline out of the monastery and into the checkout line, the argument with your partner, and the moment you want to scroll yourself numb. Mindfulness with teeth: showing up differently in how you speak, set boundaries, soothe yourself, and navigate cravings.

And yes, Buddhism shaped this framework. But it wasn't alone. Taoism, Hindu traditions, and even early Christian contemplatives taught the same core principle: Pay attention to the present moment as if your life depends on it. Because it does. Across time and geography, the teaching loops back to this: Attention is the gatekeeper of perception, mood, and meaning.

## Mindfulness as Liberation, Not Just Relaxation

Honestly, Western culture often sells mindfulness like a scented spa day for your brain. Ten minutes of breathing and soft music, and you're magically unbothered. True mindfulness is observing your mind with curiosity instead of judgment. It's noticing thoughts without feeding into shame or catastrophizing. It's not zoning out; it's tuning in.

This distinction matters: Mindfulness was designed to help humans stop suffering unnecessarily and see reality more clearly.

## Self-Compassion Versus Self-Esteem: The Buddhist Flex

Western culture spent decades pushing self-esteem as the holy grail. The early logic sounded simple: Prove yourself, achieve enough, look like you're thriving, and you'll finally feel secure. But that version of self-esteem was often conditional, built on performance, approval, or image. Which means it cracks the moment you mess up, fall short, or stop meeting whatever metric you use to justify your worth.

When self-esteem is grounded in values, community, or contribution, it can be sturdy and protective. Modern psychology leans heavily in this direction now.

But Buddhism offered something different altogether: self-compassion. The radical stance that even when you fail, struggle, or act human instead of perfect, you are still deserving of kindness. Research backs this harder than any confidence-boost slogan. A study by Kristin D. Neff and Roos Vonk, "Self-Compassion Versus Global Self-Esteem: Two Different Ways of Relating to Oneself" (2009), found that self-compassion, not contingent self-esteem, predicted long-term resilience. People high in self-compassion handled setbacks with calmer physiology, less shame, and faster recovery.

In practice, self-compassion is the friend who shows up with ice cream and zero judgment. It's the antidote to perfectionist amplification and the steady reminder that you're still enough, even when you're not "winning."

## Western Therapy's Awakening: Mindfulness Enters the Chat

While Freud was blaming your parents, other therapists were quietly borrowing from monks. By the 1970s, Jon Kabat-Zinn had launched mindfulness-based stress reduction (MBSR) to help patients manage chronic pain and stress. It worked. So well, in fact, that mindfulness walked straight into hospitals, schools, and even corporate boardrooms.

Then came mindfulness-based cognitive therapy (MBCT), which blended CBT's "challenge your thoughts" structure with mindfulness's "observe your thoughts" spaciousness. Studies showed MBCT helped prevent depressive relapses and lowered anxiety symptoms.

From there, mindfulness spread everywhere—from military resilience training and ADHD treatment to trauma therapy and even Google HQ. Sometimes helpful, sometimes hilariously misapplied (cue mandatory "mindful meetings" that are anything but).

## But Wait: The McMindfulness Problem

Not all that glitters is Zen. Critics like Ronald Purser use the term "McMindfulness" to suggest the way corporations co-opt mindfulness to squeeze more productivity out of burned-out employees. Instead of liberation, it becomes sedation: "We won't give you fair wages or fewer hours, but here's a five-minute meditation to help you cope."

Real mindfulness means freedom over sedation. It's about refusing to live on autopilot. When you learn to observe your thoughts instead of blindly acting from them, you start to notice the invisible scripts that run your life: Perform to be worthy, overextend to be liked, chase achievement to feel safe, keep the peace even when it costs you.

That internal awareness naturally spills outward.

Mindfulness trains you to pause before you comply, to question whether a demand, habit, relationship, or cultural expectation actually aligns with your values. It's harder to be manipulated by urgency, perfectionism, or external pressure when you can see how those forces land in your body and hijack your thinking. Nervous system calm gives you clarity to tell the difference between someone else's agenda and your actual needs.

In that sense, mindfulness is subversive. It breaks the trance of "should." It creates the mental space to ask better questions:

- Does this expectation serve me?
- Is this obligation aligned with my values?
- Do I want this because it's true for me or because I've been trained to want it?

That's not pacification. That's psychological sovereignty.

## A Stoic Meets the Buddha: A Fusion Practice

Want to work a tag team of East and West on your inner experience? Try this hybrid move:

1. Catch the thought. ("I'm screwing this up.")
2. Apply mindfulness. Observe the thought without judgment. Breathe.
3. Ask the Stoic question: Is this in my control?
4. Redirect. Choose a small, useful next step.

It's part Marcus Aurelius, part Buddha, part brain science and 100% a nervous system win.

## Final Thought: Your Brain, Buddha, and Balance

You can honor the science and the soul. Mindfulness isn't just for monks; it's for the anxious, the tired, the burned-out. It's for anyone ready to stop fighting their brain and start befriending it.

One breath. One thought. One act of compassion at a time. That's the East-meets-West remix.

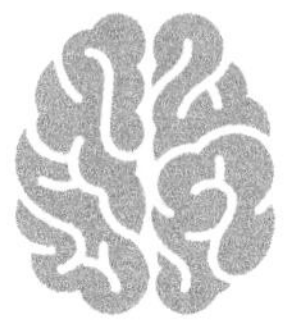



# TL;DR, DO THIS NOW, AND CLINICAL CUES

## ☑ TL;DR

- Buddhism was running the mindfulness game centuries before it became a wellness hashtag.
- The Four Noble Truths remind us that suffering is part of life, craving and clinging make it worse, and mindfulness (via the Eightfold Path) offers freedom.
- Mindfulness means liberation, not just relaxation.
- Self-compassion > self-esteem. Kindness to yourself is more resilient than chasing constant achievement.
- Western psychology caught up late but blended CBT and mindfulness into tools like MBSR and MBCT, which are science and spirituality working in tandem.

- East and West together give us both the soul and the structure: mindfulness as both ancient wisdom and modern mental health tech.

## ☑ Do This Now

1. Swap self-esteem goals ("I'll feel good when I succeed.") for self-compassion practices ("I'm kind to myself even when I struggle.").
2. Try a one-minute "observe without judgment" pause: Notice your thoughts, name them, and let them pass without needing to fix them.
3. When you feel overwhelmed, ask yourself, "Is this craving, clinging, or catastrophizing?" Labeling it is the first step in loosening its grip.
4. Blend East and West: Pick one CBT-style tool (like thought challenging) and one mindfulness tool (like breath awareness), and use them together this week.
5. Remember: Mindfulness is a way of relating to your whole messy, busy, beautiful life and not just quiet moments.

## ☑ Clinical Cues

### ▤ Heart Rate Variability (HRV)

**Why it matters:** HRV is basically your nervous system's pulse on resilience. Higher HRV means you can shift out of fight-or-flight mode instead of living mentally clenched.

Mindfulness consistently raises HRV by strengthening vagal tone and reducing sympathetic overdrive. More flexibility in your entire stress response, less white-knuckled survival mode.

## Cortisol Rhythm (especially the morning cortisol rise)

**Why it matters:** Chronic stress, perfectionism, and non-stop internal pressure distort cortisol patterns. That usually shows up as flat, sluggish mornings or wired, restless evenings. Mindfulness reduces perceived threat load and improves emotional appraisal, which aligns the cortisol curves back toward healthy: a strong rise in the morning, a calm decline at night. Sleep, mood, energy, and clarity all benefit.

## Inflammation Markers (hs-CRP, IL-6, TNF-α)

**Why it matters:** Your brain doesn't just "feel" stress. It broadcasts it. Chronic psychological strain elevates inflammatory cytokines, which are linked to fatigue, depression, anxiety, and metabolic disruption. Studies show mindfulness practices lower inflammatory signaling, especially in chronically stressed adults. Less internal fire, more emotional and physical steadiness.

### ▧ Neuroplasticity via Brain Imaging (fMRI)

**Why it matters:** This is the most undeniable evidence of all. Functional MRI scans repeatedly show that mindfulness reshapes the brain's architecture:

- Decreased default mode network activity (less self-criticism and rumination)
- Thicker prefrontal cortex (better emotional regulation, impulse control, and decision-making)
- Smaller, quieter amygdala (less panic-trigger reactivity)

This isn't visualization, "manifesting," or wishful thinking. It's neural remodeling.

### ▧ Salivary Immunoglobulin A (sIgA)

**Why it matters:** Chanting, breathwork, and mindful presence can increase sIgA levels, strengthening the gut immune barrier. Translation: better defense against infections, calmer digestion, and improved systemic resilience. When Eastern practices boost Western biomarkers, you know the bridge is real.

These aren't "perfect numbers."

They aren't personality labels.

They're biological breadcrumbs that track whether your stress circuits are loosening their grip.

None of these markers live in isolation. But when HRV rises, cortisol rhythms stabilize, inflammation quiets, neural rewiring shows up on scans, and immune markers improve?

That's your inner world remodeling itself.

Mindfulness is measurable recalibration, not escape.

## ☑ Moving On

We've traveled from Stoic chariots to Buddhist breathwork, from Harvard MRI scans to the ancient Eightfold Path, and the take-away is simple: Mindfulness works because it's both timeless and adaptable. It's philosophy, therapy, and neuroscience rolled into one. Now that we've explored how these pieces fit together, let's zoom out. In the next chapter, we'll recap everything you've learned in Part 5, so you can see the full picture of how mindfulness helps your brain, body, and nervous system find calm in a chaotic world.

# PART 5 RECAP

Mindfulness is one of the most direct ways to restore load capacity without changing a single external circumstance. When you practice mindfulness, you're literally training your nervous system to downshift out of threat mode, reducing the constant drain of vigilance, rumination, and emotional reactivity that depletes your capacity. Your Clinical Cues that mindfulness is increasing your load capacity include: more space between stimulus and response, less catastrophic thinking under stress, improved sleep quality, and feeling less hijacked by your emotions. The biological markers track with this too: HRV increases (more nervous system flexibility), cortisol curves normalize (better stress regulation), inflammation markers drop (less systemic load), and brain imaging shows actual structural changes (thicker prefrontal cortex, quieter amygdala). Mindfulness increases your capacity to meet hard things without depleting your reserves. That's the difference between surviving and having bandwidth left over to actually live.

Let's tie the threads together:

## What We've Learned

- **Mindfulness isn't a cult.** It's not robes, candles, or groupthink; it's training your brain to notice instead of react. Skepticism is healthy; avoidance isn't.
- **Your brain changes when you practice.** MRI scans prove it: The prefrontal cortex thickens (better decisions), the amygdala shrinks (less panic), the hippocampus

strengthens (more memory). Forget mysticism; mindfulness is neurological weightlifting, pure and simple.

- **The DMN is malleable.** That background station in your head that loops "You're failing"? With mindfulness, journaling, and intentional habits, you can literally change the channel. Neuroplasticity is your superpower.

- **You don't need a retreat; you need reps.** One mindful breath before your inbox. One STOP method during a spiral. One mindful walk instead of doomscrolling.

- **Stoics and Buddhists were saying the same thing in different accents.** Marcus Aurelius told us to focus only on what's in our control. The Buddha told us craving and clinging create suffering. Put them together, and you get the ultimate mental health power couple, coaching you to detach wisely, observe kindly, and act intentionally.

- **Mindfulness has East and West credibility.** Buddhism gave us the roots. Jon Kabat-Zinn brought it into hospitals. Now therapists, neuroscientists, and even skeptics can agree, it works.

- **Beware of "McMindfulness."** If a company offers breathing exercises instead of humane workloads, call it what it is: sedation, not liberation. Mindfulness should free you, not just make you more productive while you quietly burn out.

- **Self-compassion beats self-esteem.** Winning feels great until you don't win. Self-compassion carries you through the mess, calms your nervous system, and helps you bounce back faster.

## Why It Matters

Because life isn't getting quieter anytime soon. Your phone will keep buzzing. Stress will remain. The world will stay chaotic. But your response to it can change.

That's what mindfulness offers: a nervous system that can downshift out of panic, a brain that knows how to spot its own spirals, and a heart that doesn't abandon itself in the process.

This is about meeting reality with presence, strength, and clarity. And that's the kind of resilience you can take into any room, any job, any relationship, any storm.

# PART 6

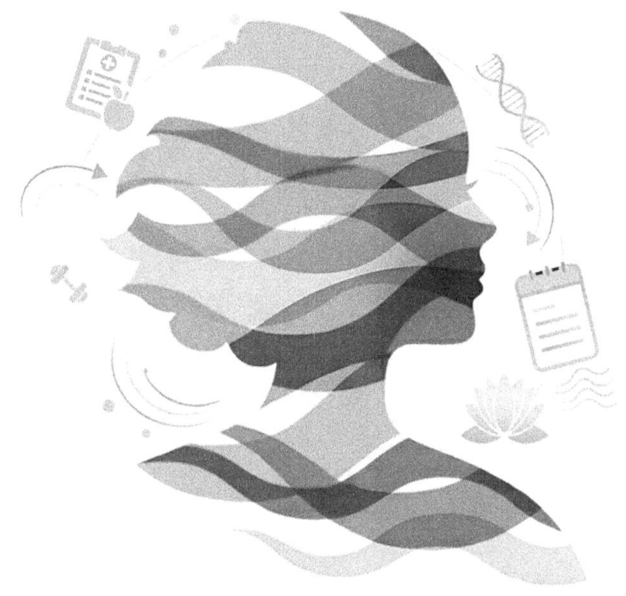

# DO SOMETHING USELESS: THE LIFE-SAVING MAGIC OF HOBBIES

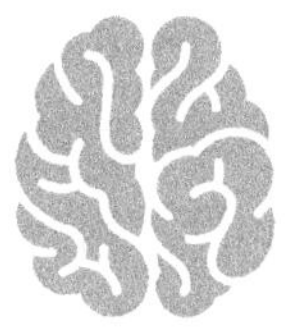



# CHAPTER 23

# THE NEUROSCIENCE OF F*CKING AROUND (AND FINDING PEACE)

You've been lied to. Somewhere along the way, we were sold the idea that every waking moment has to be productive and that if you're not working, you should be "working on yourself". Almost that fun is only acceptable if it's secretly a side hustle. Rest? That's a luxury reserved for people who've earned it by grinding themselves into the ground first. Your brain is an organism, not a machine. You're a human, not a to-do list. Constant productivity is a fast-track ticket to burnout, not a badge of honor.

Question: How's that been working out for you? Because chances are, your tired, overstimulated mind has quietly been begging for a break. Not the crash-into-the-couch kind, but the kind of break that actually restores you.

This is where hobbies come in. Remember hobbies? The things you do just because they bring you joy, not because they get you ahead. The so-called "pointless" activities that, truth bomb, are anything but. Hobbies reclaim your sanity in a world that worships the grind. They are essential. They are healing. And yes, they are absolutely allowed. This chapter is your permission slip (cosigned by science) to do something utterly useless, simply for the joy of it, and in doing so, give your brain exactly what it needs to function, flourish, and maybe even have a little fun for once.

## Evolution Wired You for Play

It turns out, play is wired into us as a survival mechanism. Jaak Panksepp, the neuroscientist who mapped the brain's play circuitry, argued that play is as essential as sleep or hunger for mammalian nervous systems. Stuart Brown, author of *Play: How It Shapes the Brain, Opens the Imagination, and Invigorates the Soul,* took those findings further by showing that the absence of play in adulthood is linked to rigidity, emotional volatility, and even aggression. What does that mean? Your hobbies are your nervous system's evolutionary repair kit. Play keeps your stress response flexible instead of brittle. Adult play = regulation.

## Flow State: The Brain's Reset Button

Let's talk science. Ever heard of a "flow state"? It's that magical zone where you're so into what you're doing, everything else just fades away. Time disappears, stress vanishes, and all that matters is the thing in front of you. Flow is legit neuroscience, thanks to psychologist Mihaly Csikszentmihalyi (yep, impossible to pronounce, but stay with me) spent decades studying this phenomenon and mapped it as a measurable brain state.

When you hit flow, your brain releases a potent mix of feel-good chemicals: dopamine, norepinephrine, and your own natural endocannabinoids. (Yes, your brain has its own dispensary.) These molecules regulate mood, reduce pain, and quiet stress. They're why knitting, drumming, painting, skateboarding, or even perfecting your latte art can feel like therapy.

Flow makes you feel good in the moment and trains your nervous system for resilience. Research shows it acts like stress inoculation. The more often you practice slipping into flow, the faster your brain recovers from stress outside of it. Flow is like emotional Pilates, training your nervous system to bounce back stronger.

## Trauma, Hobbies, and Nervous System Repair

If you've lived through trauma, your nervous system might operate in survival mode more often than it needs to: jumpy, on alert, and chronically tense. This is where hobbies become low-stakes, high-reward therapy. Polyvagal theory, developed by Stephen Porges, explains it like this: Safe play activates your vagus nerve's ventral branch, the part of your nervous system that's wired for connection and safety, and you enter a ventral vagal state. When you lose yourself in painting, drumming, gardening, or even building Legos castles, your body reads it as proof: "I am safe now."

This is why trauma therapists often prescribe "structured play" for adults: crocheting, pottery, music, improv. This is about retraining your nervous system to believe life can be more than scanning for danger.

## The Hustle Culture Hobby Hijack

Here's the dark side: We live in a culture that can't leave hobbies alone. The moment you start baking bread, someone asks if you're selling sourdough on Etsy. You learn to knit, and suddenly it's "Have you considered opening an Instagram shop?"

Hustle culture ruins hobbies by trying to monetize them. But hobbies lose their magic the moment they have to justify themselves. Your watercolor painting doesn't have to hang in a gallery. Your Dungeons & Dragons campaign doesn't need a Twitch channel. The whole point is that it's gloriously useless.

Protect your hobbies from capitalism. They're one of the last sacred spaces where you get to be a human being, not a human resource.

## Cortisol, Community, and Identity

Of course, it's not just brain chemistry in the moment. Hobbies have long-term mental health benefits too:

- Cortisol drop: Enjoyable activities lower chronic stress hormones. Your body shifts from fight-or-flight mode into rest-and-digest mode.

- Neuroplasticity: Learning a new skill literally rewires your brain. [Draganski et al. (2006)]
- Identity: Hobbies give you a self beyond your roles as worker, parent, partner. They remind you that you're allowed to exist outside of usefulness.
- Community: Trivia nights, pottery studios, cosplay conventions, knitting circles, or even Discord servers. Hobbies create belonging. And connection is one of the strongest predictors of long-term health. [Holt-Lunstad et al. (2010)]

## My Brain on Axe Throwing

And sometimes, hobbies look a little less like calm journaling and a little more like hurling sharp objects.

So there I was, standing in front of a giant wooden bullseye, holding an axe that was way heavier than I expected, and questioning every life choice that led me here. "Just picture your stress on the target," the instructor said. And let me tell you, there was plenty of material.

First throw? Total flop. Second throw? Closer. Third throw? Dead center. Victory. Pure, chaotic, stress-melting victory.

I didn't walk out of there thinking I'd found my new career as a lumberjack. For that hour, my brain focused on one thing: hitting the target. I was present. Fierce. Alive.

Moral of the story? Sometimes your nervous system needs to throw an axe and whisper, "Take that, patriarchy."

## Bottom Line

Hobbies aren't breaks from life; they *are* life. They light up your endocannabinoid system, reset your default mode network, lower cortisol, and remind you who you are outside of what you produce.

Your skill level doesn't matter. Your knitting can look like spaghetti; your brain gets the benefit anyway.

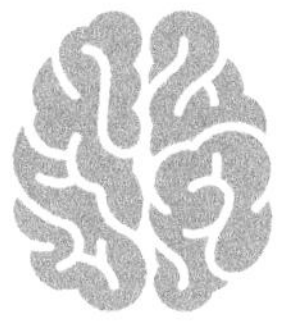



# TL;DR, DO THIS NOW, AND CLINICAL CUES

## ☑ TL;DR

- Your brain is an organism that needs play, not a productivity machine.
- Hobbies trigger flow states, lower cortisol, and release natural chill chemicals.
- Safe play rewires the nervous system toward safety, so it's especially beneficial for trauma survivors.
- Protect your joy from hustle culture. Your hobbies exist for pleasure, not performance.
- Being alive matters more than being good.

## ☑ **Do This Now**

Pick one hobby you've been secretly curious about, and give your-self *permission to suck.* Schedule twenty guilt-free minutes this week to try it. That's it. Your nervous system will thank you.

## ☑ **Clinical Cues**

### ▪ **Prolactin (serum)**

- Normal: ~4–23 ng/mL (Adult women, may vary slightly by lab and menstrual phase.)

**Why it matters:** Chronic stress elevates prolactin, which sup-presses dopamine—your joy, motivation, reward, and desire circuitry. When you stay locked in survival-mode productivity, prolactin often creeps upward. Hobbies, novelty, laughter, and nonproductive pleasure lower stress load and help prolactin normalize. When prolactin trends down through joy, sponta-neity, and "pointless" play, your emotional spark comes back online.

**Translation:** Your brain becomes more lit up, curious, playful, and self-directed because you stopped living like you're being graded.

## ▦ High-Sensitivity C-Reactive Protein (hs-CRP)

- Optimal: <1.0 mg/L
- Mild systemic inflammation: 1–3 mg/L
- High inflammation: >3 mg/L

**Why it matters:** Overwork, perfectionism, emotional suppression, chronic vigilance, and "hyperfunctional woman syndrome" raise inflammatory molecules. That inflammation shows up as fatigue, irritability, brain fog, achy tension, and more reactive stress responses.

Research shows play, social enjoyment, rest, and flow experiences reduce inflammatory tone, and hs-CRP is one of the most reliable blood markers to track the shift.

**Translation:** The more you let yourself be human—laughing, creating, exploring, messing around—the quieter your systemic inflammation gets.

## ▦ Estradiol (E2)

Typical reference ranges for menstruating women:

- Follicular phase: ~30–120 pg/mL
- Ovulation peak: up to ~100–400 pg/mL
- Luteal phase: ~50–250 pg/mL

(Ranges vary slightly by lab, but the physiology is universal.)

**Why it matters:** Estradiol takes a hit when the body lives in "survive, not thrive" mode. Chronic stress blunts ovarian signaling through the brain's stress hormone pathways. Low estradiol shows up as anxiety, irritability, low motivation, poor recovery, flat mood, and feeling disconnected from joy. Play, creativity, pleasure, and safe novelty reactivate parasympathetic tone and HPA–HPG dialogue, supporting healthier hormonal rhythms.

**Translation:** When you stop living like a robot, your chemistry remembers you're human.

### ▪ Vitamin D (25-OH)

- Insufficient: <30 ng/mL
- Optimal for mental health, immune resilience, and mood regulation: ~50–70 ng/mL

(Some endocrine panels allow up to 80 ng/mL as "optimal," but 50–70 ng/mL is most widely accepted.)

**Why it matters:** Vitamin D is tied to mood, neuroplasticity, immunity, inflammation, and stress recovery. Outdoor hobbies, sunlight, embodied movement, and social play naturally support vitamin D synthesis. Low levels correlate with depressive mood, low energy, irritability, and stress sensitivity. When vitamin D climbs into the optimal range, most women report steadier mood, better resilience, and more "aliveness."

**Translation:** Sun-drenched joy counts as therapy. And it shows up in your labs.

## ☑ Moving On

Hobbies are medicine. But what if you don't know what yours are? Or worse, you think you don't have any? In the next chapter, we'll build you a menu of options, from cozy solo crafts to adrenaline-fueled chaos, so you can find the ones that light up your brain.

Because f*ck around long enough, and you'll find the peace you've been missing.

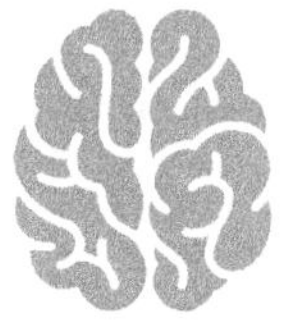



# CHAPTER 24

# CALM YOUR CHAOS: MINDFUL HOBBIES FOR THE ANXIOUS BRAIN

Let's get something straight: Your brain is tired because we live in a world that never shuts up. Between constant screen time, background noise, and the endless pressure to multitask, your nervous system is being zapped with dopamine jolts it was never built to handle. Every ping, scroll, and "just one more task" feels rewarding in the moment but eventually leaves you overstimulated, wired, and worn out.

This goes beyond typical tiredness. You're too wound-up to rest, too depleted to function. Your to-do list is anxious. Your thoughts feel like tornadoes. And here's the good news: Gentle, mindful hobbies can reset your baseline. They're survival skills for a nervous system that's forgotten how to breathe.

## The Science of Slow

Here's why slow, mindful hobbies work:

- Polyvagal reset: Rhythmic activities (knitting, coloring, walking) stimulate the vagus nerve, shifting you out of fight-or-flight mode and into rest-and-digest mode.
- Dopamine balance: Unlike the spiky highs of social media, calm hobbies give you steady, sustainable dopamine hits, the kind your brain can actually regulate.
- DMN downshift: Remember the default mode network? Hobbies like gardening and puzzles quiet its anxious loops, letting your mind wander in restorative ways.

These are structural shifts. They show your body and brain relearning how to downshift without spiraling.

## Knitting, Gardening, and Legos Therapy

Take knitting. It looks like grandma's pastime, but neurologically? It's rhythmic, meditative, and grounding. The gentle click of needles engages sensorimotor pathways, slows your heart rate, and lowers cortisol. Your brain, overstimulated by modern life, finally has a beat it can rest against.

Or gardening. Sure, the tomatoes are one perk, but more than that, you'll get a sensory immersion that connects you to something bigger. Touching soil, smelling herbs, watching life grow, it literally grounds you. Studies show even short doses of green space lower stress hormones and boost mood. Plus, nothing hits quite like the thrill of keeping something alive besides yourself.

Not into dirt or yarn? Try puzzles, Legos, or model building. These give your brain an activity that's concrete, manageable, and low stakes. Problem-solving without panic. Concentration without cortisol. The opposite of doomscrolling.

## When Art and Music Become Medicine

Coloring, painting, doodling: These are scientifically validated mindfulness practices. When you focus on lines and colors, your stress-driven brain finally has a safe landing strip. That's why adult coloring books blew up: They work.

Photography is another gem. Looking through a lens forces you to notice light, detail, and texture. Suddenly, you're seeing beauty in a world your stressed-out brain usually rushes past. That's mindfulness with a shutter click.

Music belongs here too. Whether you're playing, singing, or just listening deeply, music activates emotional regulation centers and syncs your brain's rhythms. It's why one song can make you cry, dance, or feel like yourself again in seconds.

## From Frazzled to Flow

I'll never forget the week I was so fried I couldn't read a single sentence without reflexively opening another tab and doomscrolling. Out of desperation, I picked up a half-finished puzzle. At first it felt pointless. But twenty minutes later, I realized I hadn't checked my phone once. My chest felt lighter. The loop in my head, gone. That puzzle gave my brain a pocket of peace. Sometimes that's the first domino.

## Cultural Permission Slip

Here's the thing: Kids are encouraged to color, sing, garden, and play. Adults? We're told those same activities are "wasting time." That's nonsense. Somewhere along the way, we replaced joy with productivity and forgot that play is how humans regulate. Calm hobbies = medicine.

And especially for women, this is radical. Too often, our identities get swallowed by our roles: caretaker, professional, fixer of all things. Gentle hobbies give you something that's just yours. A thread back to yourself.

## When Calm Isn't Enough

Sometimes your nervous system needs activation, not calm. Sometimes your nervous system is flatlined and too numb for knitting, too drained for gardening. That's when you need hobbies that wake you back up. The kind that bring color, energy, and aliveness back to your body.

A salsa class where you're tripping over your own feet. Axe throwing. Rock climbing just high enough to make your legs shake. Roller-skating around the neighborhood. Belly laughing through improv. Learning drums and feeling the vibration through your ribs. Even a beginner hip-hop class where you look ridiculous but feel deliciously awake.

Those are invitations back into your body, not escapes.

## The Point Is: Just Show Up

Whether you're buzzing with anxiety or burnt out into numbness, there's a hobby out there that can meet you. No metrics. No monetization. No gold stars. Just a chance to reclaim your nervous system, one small practice at a time.

Because peace isn't inherited; it's a skill. And hobbies are how you practice.

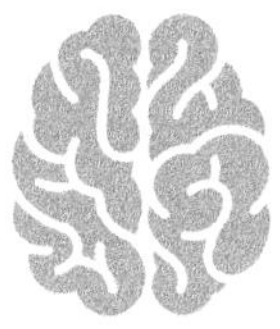



# TL;DR, DO THIS NOW, AND CLINICAL CUES

## ☑ TL;DR

Your brain is fried because the modern world overstimulates you 24/7. Calm, mindful hobbies are the antidote. They reset your nervous system, balance your dopamine, and quiet the anxious loops in your default mode network.

## ☑ Do This Now

Pick one:

- 🧶 Rhythmic calm: Try five minutes of knitting, coloring, or doodling. Repetition = nervous system reset.

- 🪴 Ground in green: Step outside, touch some plants, breathe the air. Gardening = cortisol killer.
- 🧩 Low-stakes focus: Start a puzzle, Legos build, or model. Win small, calm big.
- 🎶 Music medicine: Put on one song, and really listen. Bonus points if you sing or dance along.
- 🚶 Reset walk: Take a ten-minute stroll (no phone). Notice sights, sounds, steps.

*Rules of Engagement*

1. You don't have to be good at it.
2. You don't have to post about it.
3. You don't have to explain it.

Just show up. Let your brain exhale.

## ☑ Clinical Cues

### ▪ DHEA-S (serum)

- Reference: ~35–430 µg/dL
- Optimal: ~200–350 µg/dL

**Why it matters:** DHEA is the nervous system's biological shock absorber. Chronic mental overload, perfectionism, and nonstop "doing mode" drain it.

Low DHEA = low resilience: brain fog, depleted motivation, emotional fragility.

Gentle hobbies, sensory immersion, and time spent in flow reverse that drop. When DHEA-S rises toward the optimal window, it's biochemical evidence that your system is shifting out of threat mode and back toward vitality.

**Translation:** A healthier DHEA-S level is your body saying, "I'm safe enough to rebuild."

## Homocysteine (serum)

- Reference: 5–15 µmol/L
- Optimal for brain and mood regulation: 6–9 µmol/L

**Why it matters:** Homocysteine reveals nervous system inflammation, not just cardiovascular risk. It spikes when the nervous system is inflamed, tightly wound, or running on adrenaline. Elevated levels are linked to irritability, anxiety, cognitive rigidity, and slower emotional repair.

Slow, rhythmic hobbies lower homocysteine by improving metabolic methylation, calming inflammatory pathways, and restoring neurochemical equilibrium.

**Translation:** When homocysteine drops below 9, your brain is less inflamed, thinking is clearer, and emotional recovery runs smoother.

### ▪ Blood Lactate (serum)

- Reference (fasting): ~0.5–2.2 mmol/L
- Optimal nervous system regulation: <1.5 mmol/L

**Why it matters:** Lactate reveals nervous system state beyond fitness tracking. When resting lactate runs high, it signals that the nervous system is stuck in high gear even at baseline. It's physiology's version of "I can't shut my brain off."

Mindful hobbies lower lactate by reducing sympathetic drive, improving oxygen utilization, and shifting metabolism away from stress-burn.

When lactate drops into the optimal zone, it's evidence that your system is finally gliding instead of grinding.

**Translation:** Lower lactate = the chemistry of "I actually feel calm" rather than "I'm pretending to be calm."

### ▪ Dopamine Beta-Hydroxylase (DBH) Activity (plasma or serum)

- Reference activity: ~40–80 U/L
(Ranges vary slightly by lab, but this is the standard reference band.)
- Optimal for balanced neuro-arousal: mid-range, ~50–65 U/L

**Why it matters:** DBH is the enzyme that converts dopamine into norepinephrine.

If activity is too high, dopamine drains fast and anxiety chemistry dominates: restlessness, tension, sensory overload, doomscroll urgency, perfectionist drive.

If DBH is too low, dopamine bottlenecks, and you feel flat, unmotivated, and emotionally muted.

When hobbies invite novelty, rhythm, flow, and pleasure, DBH moderates toward mid-range balance.

You metabolize dopamine steadily instead of burning it out.

Norepinephrine quiets down from siren mode into focus and calm.

**Translation:** DBH in the sweet spot is biochemical proof that you're no longer running life on adrenaline.

## ☑ Moving On

But here's the snag: Even with all this science and soul behind hobbies, most of us still don't do them. Why? Because of the lies we tell ourselves: "I don't have time." "I'm not good at anything." "It's selfish." These stories aren't harmless; they're the quiet saboteurs keeping you stuck in burnout. In the next chapter, we're going to call them out, dismantle them one by one, and finally give you permission to do something "useless" without the guilt.

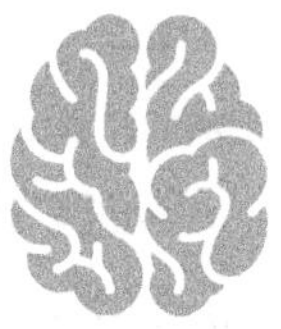



# CHAPTER 25

# THE HOBBY LIES WE TELL OURSELVES (AND WHY THEY'RE RUINING US)

Let's have a brutally honest moment, just you and me. You've probably convinced yourself at some point that hobbies are a "nice idea" for people who have less going on than you. Maybe you've thought, *I don't have time for that,* or *I wouldn't even know what to do,* or *I'd feel guilty taking time for myself.*

These thoughts are toxic, keeping you stuck in a cycle of burnout, self-neglect, and low-key resentment. The lies we tell ourselves about why we can't do something just for fun? They're the same lies that keep us mentally and emotionally exhausted. And it's time to call BS.

## Lie #1: *I don't have time.*

Oh really? You have time to scroll Instagram for forty-five minutes while you "unwind," but you don't have fifteen minutes to do something that actually restores you? Let's break this down. The average adult in developed countries spends more than two hours a day on social media (Statista, 2023). That's 730 hours a year. Let that sink in. That's nearly a month, gone.

It's not just about minutes on the clock. Psychologists like Ashley Whillans talk about *time affluence,* the feeling of having enough time for what matters. People who deliberately carve out small moments for leisure report far higher life satisfaction, even if they're busy. In other words, you don't need hours. You need permission.

## Lie #2: *I'm not good at anything.*

You are not required to be "good" at something to enjoy it. That's a myth born from a culture obsessed with outcomes. We've been taught to only value activities if they produce results, accolades, or income. But hobbies don't exist to prove your worth. They exist to nourish your soul.

Being a beginner is one of the healthiest things you can do. Trying something awkward, uncertain, even messy is exactly what your brain craves. Neuroscience shows us that learning new skills increases gray matter density in the brain [Draganski et al. (2006)], improves memory, and enhances cognitive flexibility. Your brain thrives when you let yourself stumble through something new.

Nobody gets inspired by watching flawless execution; they get inspired by watching people *try*. When you fail and laugh and keep going, you're showing that joy exists independent of skill.

## Lie #3: *It's indulgent. I should be doing something useful.*

This one's the most dangerous because it hides under the guise of responsibility. If you're constantly drained, constantly giving, constantly running on empty, how exactly are you supposed to show up fully in any part of your life?

Hobbies aren't indulgent. They're essential. Research in the *Journal of Occupational Health Psychology* found that engaging in leisure activities reduces emotional exhaustion, improves well-being, and increases life satisfaction. [Sonnentag (2001)] In other words, doing something "pointless" actually makes you more effective everywhere else.

## Bonus Trap: The Hustle Culture Lie

Even when we do pick up hobbies, hustle culture whispers, "Monetize it." Love painting? "Sell on Etsy." Like running? "Train for a sponsored marathon." Into photography? "Better start a side business."

The rebellion: The second you attach pressure, the mental health benefits vanish. A hobby that exists only to soothe, energize, and delight you is revolutionary.

## The Neuroscience of Guilt-Free Play

Still feel guilty? Let's make this biological. Your brain *needs* "useless" play. Downtime consolidates memory, restores focus, lowers cortisol, and activates the default mode network in healthy, creative ways. Without it, your brain fries out. With it, you think better, feel better, and function better.

Hobbies fuel productivity. They don't steal from it; they feed it. They give you back the mental clarity to enjoy your family, career, and goals.

## The Truth You Can't Ignore

Your brain deserves more than just work and survival. You are here for more than grinding through life, ticking boxes, and chasing goals until you collapse. Hobbies are a rebellion against that.

They are how you take back your time, your energy, and your joy. They're a middle finger to burnout culture and a love letter to your most authentic self.

So go ahead: Do something useless. On purpose. Let it be messy. Let it be small. Let it be yours. And in that space, watch how your world begins to shift.

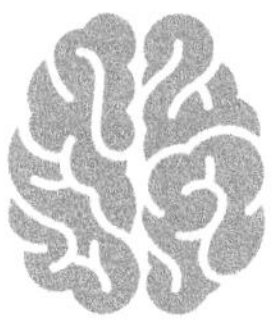



# TL;DR, DO THIS NOW, AND CLINICAL CUES

## ☑ TL;DR

Here's what you've been telling yourself:

- "I don't have time."
- "I'm not good at anything."
- "It's indulgent."
- "I should monetize this."

Here's the truth:

- You *do* have time; you're just spending it on mindless scrolling.
- Beginners' brains grow stronger. Skill is irrelevant.

- Play is medicine for burnout.
- Hobbies don't need an audience or an income stream. They need *you*.

## ☑ Do This Now

1. Claim fifteen minutes. That's it. Replace one scroll session with one joy session.
2. Start messy. Pick something small: Doodle, strum, walk, bake, knit a wobbly square.
3. Keep it offline. No posting. No proving. Just play.
4. Notice the shift. Track how you feel after. Not how "good" you were.

Your hobby doesn't have to change the world. It just has to change *your* nervous system.

## ☑ Clinical Cues

### ▣ Brain-Derived Neurotrophic Factor (BDNF, serum)

- Normal: ~10–30 ng/mL (Ranges vary by lab.)
- Optimal: upper half of range

**Why it matters:** BDNF is your brain's "growth signal," the molecule that helps you learn, adapt, regulate emotions, and stay mentally flexible. Low BDNF shows up in women who run on autopilot, overwork, and rarely do anything new or joyful. It looks like rigid thinking, low curiosity, repeat stress loops, flat mood.

Novelty-driven hobbies—learning guitar, painting badly, trying pottery, even fumbling through a dance class—raise BDNF. They tell your nervous system "We're safe enough to grow again." Higher BDNF = better mood, sharper memory, and a brain that isn't slowly closing in on itself.

## CoQ10 (serum, functional)

- Normal: 0.7–1.0 µg/mL
- Optimal: >1.3 µg/mL

**Why it matters:** CoQ10 is mitochondrial currency. When life becomes all grind and zero nourishment, your mitochondria downshift energy production and antioxidant defense. Low CoQ10 reads like exhaustion that coffee can't fix, emotional flatness, brain fog, and "I'm tired down to my bones."

Flow-state hobbies—puzzles, gardening, knitting, music— boost parasympathetic tone, sleep quality, vascular health, and oxygenation. Those changes raise CoQ10 and restore cellular energy. Translation: When you bring joy back into your life, your mitochondria stop waving the white flag.

## Vitamin B6 (P5P, plasma)

- Normal: 5–50 mcg/L
- Optimal: 20–50 mcg/L

**Why it matters:** B6 is a cofactor for serotonin and dopamine synthesis, which means it's your biochemical bridge from play to good mood. Chronic stress and perfectionism burn through B6 fast and the body uses it up trying to keep cortisol in check.

Low B6 looks like irritability, low motivation, emotional volatility, PMS mood shifts, cravings, and that "I don't enjoy anything anymore" numbness.

Hobbies help restore B6 by improving digestion, vagal tone, and nervous system calm. When you reintroduce joy, play, and restorative slowness into your life, B6 rebounds, and suddenly your brain remembers what pleasure feels like.

## Moving On

We've learned that hobbies make your life better on every level. Here's the bigger picture: Reclaiming joy in "pointless" things extends beyond hobbies. It's about rewriting your relationship to rest, energy, and survival. And if hobbies are how you reclaim the day, sleep is how you reclaim the night.

So let's talk about that other "optional luxury" you've been skipping: sleep. Because guess what? It's not optional.

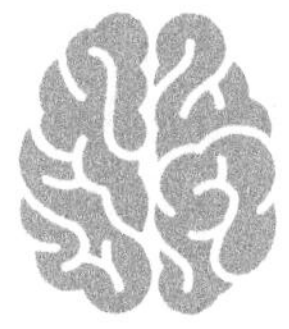



# CHAPTER 26

# SLEEP? NEVER HEARD OF HER

Sleep is foundational. It's your nervous system's reset button, your brain's garbage disposal, and your emotional-regulation software update, all in one.

And yet most of us treat sleep like that flaky friend who always bails. We know we need her, but we keep swiping right on caffeine at 4 p.m., blue light until midnight, and stress spirals that make our brains feel like late-night cable reruns. Cute.

If you're anxious, depressed, burned out, or just tired of life, sleep is the first thing to fix.

## Why Sleep Matters (And Why It Feels So Impossible)

When you cut sleep short or get poor-quality rest, your amygdala goes into full *Real Housewives* mode. You become more reactive, more anxious, and less rational, and your body floods with inflammation.

This is biochemical volatility, beyond typical tiredness. Long-term sleep loss leads to:

- Increased risk of depression and burnout
- Impulsivity and poor decision-making
- Weight gain and metabolic issues
- Cognitive decline and thick brain fog
- Emotional fragility (because BDNF, your brain's growth factor, tanks without sleep)

Sleep is where neuroplasticity happens. It's where your brain literally detoxes itself through the glymphatic system. It's where hormones balance, memory consolidates, and your nervous system resets. Miss it, and you're not just tired, you're mentally and physically compromised.

## Your Brain's Load Capacity: Why Some Days Break You and Others Don't

Every woman has a biological capacity for stress. It isn't fixed, it isn't emotional fragility, and it isn't about discipline. It's determined by how resourced your brain and body are when life applies pressure. Sleep depth, micronutrient sufficiency, glucose stability, inflammation exposure, and hormonal balance all raise or lower your internal bandwidth. When those foundations are depleted, stress feels sharper, small setbacks feel threatening, and emotional regulation becomes harder because your system is underfueled and undersupported.

You can think of load capacity in three layers:

**Layer 1: Physiological Foundation**

This is the biochemical floor your brain stands on.

Omega-3 status, ferritin and iron reserves, B vitamins, magnesium, vitamin D, sleep architecture, metabolic flexibility, and mitochondrial efficiency all influence how steady and resilient your nervous system feels. When these are strong, you have biochemical padding. When they're low, you're emotionally brittle and easier to overload.

**Layer 2: Modulators**

Hormones, inflammation, immune tone, menstrual phase, stress history, and current inflammatory triggers sit here. They tilt your baseline up or down on any given week. This is why luteal shifts, sleep loss, iron dips, or high-glycemic eating change your stress tolerance, mood stability, cravings, cognition, and anxiety responsiveness, even when "nothing dramatic" is happening around you.

**Layer 3: Expression Layer**

This is what you feel and how you act: mood, irritability, urgency, rumination, panic, emotional withdrawal, overreaction, or that sense that everything is too much. They're reflections of your foundation and modulators. When the base layers are fueled and supported, your thoughts are more flexible, your emotions are less explosive, and your inner world feels steadier and kinder.

**Here's the important part:**

Your brain can only respond to stress at the level your foundation and modulators allow. If sleep is shallow, inflammation is high, ferritin is low, glucose is unstable, magnesium is depleted, or hormones are shifting, your capacity shrinks. If you strengthen those variables, the same stressor that once felt unbearable becomes something you can navigate with perspective and calm.

This is why the chapters on nutrition, labs, movement, sleep, and mindfulness aren't separate wellness topics. They're levers that raise load capacity so you can handle the life you already have without feeling like your brain is betraying you.

Your nervous system needs more support than you've been taught to give it.

## Meet Your Sleep Squad (And Sleep Saboteurs)
### Who's running the night shift in your brain?

**Melatonin**

Melatonin is your brain's "lights out" announcement, not the sandman knocking you unconscious. Darkness triggers the pineal gland to release it, signaling every system to power down and switch into repair mode.

When you're glued to screens at night, overscheduled, or mentally revved, that signal shows up late or weak. Cue: wired brain, restless sleep, dragging mornings, and the classic "Why am I tired but also awake?" paradox. That's melatonin begging for a chance to do its job.

## Adenosine

Think of adenosine as sleep pressure accumulating like "brain debt" throughout the day. The more it builds, the harder your system nudges you toward rest. Caffeine blocks adenosine receptors, so you can't feel how tired you are until it wears off. When the caffeine wears off, fatigue hits like a brick. If life is nonstop stimulation, multitasking, and brain clutter, adenosine never gets a clean rhythm. End result: numbed-out exhaustion, broken sleep cues, and that zombie feeling when you finally stop moving.

## GABA

GABA is your internal dimmer switch. When it's strong, your mind feels like a quiet library: clear, calm, and focused. When it's low, every thought is a megaphone. Racing at bedtime, looping worries, mental static, irritability, and "I can't shut my brain up" nights are all classic low-GABA signatures. Rhythmic, absorbing hobbies—knitting, coloring, music, puzzles—all increase GABA tone naturally. It's brain chemistry's version of turning down the noise and breathing again.

## Cortisol

Cortisol is meant to peak in the morning, not ambush you at 3 a.m. It's your dawn alertness hormone, like internal espresso. But when stress is constant and your system is trained to stay on guard, cortisol flips its schedule. Nights become restless and brain-spinny, and mornings feel like swimming through wet cement. Slow hobbies help retrain cortisol back into daytime duty. When cortisol behaves, nights get sleepier and mornings finally start to feel human again.

## Serotonin → Melatonin Conversion

Serotonin is daytime steadiness: mood, focus, and emotional bandwidth. When night hits, your brain repurposes serotonin into melatonin, which is your biological "go to bed" signal. The pathway is straightforward:

tryptophan → 5-HTP → serotonin → N-acetylserotonin → melatonin

If serotonin is low because you never see sunlight, you're chronically stressed, understimulated, or living on low-nutrient food, melatonin can't form properly. Cue: restless sleep cycles, shallow rest, early-morning wake-ups, and mornings that feel like anesthesia hangovers. Creativity, sunlight, hobbies, and flow-state activities boost serotonin by day so your body can make melatonin at night. No serotonin, no sleep chemistry. It's that simple.

## Orexin + Histamine

Orexin and histamine are your brain's internal "stay awake and scan the horizon" chemicals. They're perfect when you need vigilance but terrible when you're trying to sleep. Chronic stress, inflammation, anxiety, or emotional overload keep them firing, which traps your nervous system in alert mode even when you're curled up in bed. Calm, absorbing hobbies quiet orexin and histamine which is the biological equivalent of telling your brain "We're safe. Shut it down." When those two ease off, sleep finally feels like sleep.

When your routine, environment, and habits send the wrong cues, this whole orchestra turns into a dubstep remix of panic and exhaustion.

## Why You Can't Sleep Even When You're Exhausted

Our biology evolved for sunrises and sunsets. Enter: modern life. Now we've got:

- 24/7 artificial light
- Endless screen time
- Doomscrolling at 1 a.m.
- Stress and cortisol spikes
- Jet-lagged circadian rhythms from irregular meals and movement

Your body is basically screaming, "What time zone is this even?!"

## The Sleep–Mental Health Feedback Loop

- Poor sleep cranks up anxiety.
- Anxiety makes it harder to sleep.
- Repeat until burnout.

Science shows sleep deprivation ramps up your amygdala and disconnects it from your prefrontal cortex, a.k.a. your adult brain.

That means less resilience, less focus, more emotional chaos. And because sleep loss lowers BDNF, you actually lose flexibility in the way your brain processes stress.

Insomnia takes your sleep and erodes your mental steadiness.

## Sleep Hygiene (But Make It Realistic)

Forget the capitalistic wellness influencer routines. These are the things that actually work:

1. Morning light. Five to ten minutes outside within thirty minutes of waking anchors your circadian clock.
2. Caffeine cutoff. After 2 p.m., it's not your friend. That 4 p.m. cold brew is why you're staring at the ceiling.
3. Screen discipline. Blue light = melatonin killer. Use filters or glasses if you can't unplug.
4. Wind-down ritual. Think dim lights, warm shower, journaling, magnesium + theanine, no doom TV.
5. Alcohol check. Sure, it knocks you out, but it shreds REM sleep and spikes nighttime cortisol.

## Supplements: Helpful, Not Magical

Supplements can nudge sleep without replacing rhythm. Think helpers, not fixes.

- L-theanine: calms the anxious brain
- Magnesium glycinate: relaxes muscles, reduces tension

- Glycine: drops core body temp, deepens REM
- PharmaGABA: great for racing thoughts
- Ashwagandha: for high nighttime cortisol
- Melatonin (low dose!): only if you struggle to fall asleep, not stay asleep

## Personalized Fixes: Choose Your Struggle

- Can't fall asleep? → Light hygiene (no blue light within two hours of bedtime), magnesium, no evening news
- Can't stay asleep? → Check blood sugar (try a small protein snack), glycine, or GABA
- Anxious before bed? → Yoga nidra or Non-Sleep Deep Rest (NSDR), gratitude journaling, L-theanine
- Waking wired at 3 a.m.? → Probably cortisol, cut sugar at dinner, consider adaptogens

## When to Call In Backup

If you've tried the basics and you're still a zombie:

- Rule out sleep apnea (especially if snoring/waking up gasping).
- Check hormones (progesterone, thyroid, estrogen, cortisol).
- Try cognitive behavioral therapy for insomnia (CBT-I), the gold standard for insomnia treatment.
- Use medications sparingly and only with supervision.

## Bottom Line

Sleep is biologically necessary. You just need to stop fighting the signals your body is already sending. Your brain is begging for repair. Your body is waiting for regulation. And you? You deserve to wake up feeling human again.

So seriously: Turn off your phone, close this book, and go to bed.

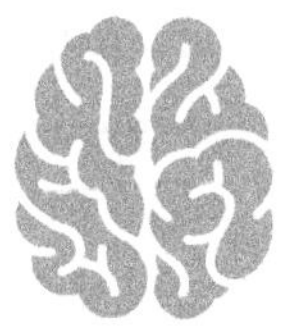



# TL;DR, DO THIS NOW, AND CLINICAL CUES

## ☑ TL;DR

Your brain can't heal, grow, or function without sleep. You don't earn it; you need it. Here's the no-BS version:

**The Big Why**

- Sleep = emotional regulation + memory consolidation + brain detox
- Skipping it = anxiety spikes, depression risk, burnout, brain fog
- Chronic loss = You're not a snail brain; you're biologically compromised.

If you wouldn't expect a laptop to run at full speed with 3% battery, don't blame yourself when sleep deprivation makes your mind lag.

## ☑ Do This Now

### Your Nonnegotiables

- Morning light: Five to ten minutes outside ASAP after waking
- Caffeine cutoff: None after 2 p.m. (yes, even "just one espresso")
- Digital dimmer: Screens wreck melatonin; filter them or shut them down.
- Wind-down routine: Give your body consistent cues like dim lights, stretching, journaling, magnesium.
- Alcohol reality check: Knocks you out, wrecks REM. Sedation ≠ sleep.

### Red Flags (Get Support If . . .)

- Loud snoring, gasping, or choking → check for sleep apnea
- Weeks of insomnia despite basics → CBT-I
- Constant exhaustion → test hormones, thyroid, cortisol

### Pep Talk

Your rest is already yours. Reclaim it. Start tonight.

## ☑ Clinical Cues

*(Note: Some of these biomarkers don't have fixed reference ranges. They're interpreted by pattern, trend, and alignment with symptoms rather than by a single number. Functional clinicians look at curve shape, direction of change, and whether values normalize as sleep and recovery improve.)*

### ▪ Melatonin (salivary or urinary, functional panel)

Melatonin doesn't have a universal "normal range," because levels shift based on when you test, how you test, and how much light you've been living under. What matters is the nightly arc: Melatonin should rise sharply after dark, peak between 2 and 4 a.m., and then taper toward morning. Women with chronic insomnia, late-night screen habits, or circadian disruption often show a flattened pattern: low rise and low peak, which usually lines up with narrative clues like "wired at night, dead in the morning."

### ▪ 24-Hour Cortisol Curve (salivary or urinary mapping)

A single cortisol blood draw tells you almost nothing about your stress rhythm. Cortisol is read as a four-point arc across the day, not a static number. A healthy curve spikes soon after waking, slopes steadily downward, and bottoms out at night. When the shape inverts, low in the morning, too high at night, you usually see the lived experience that matches it: exhausted on waking, wired late, and scrolling at 1 a.m. The curve is the story.

### ■ IGF-1 (serum)

IGF-1 finally gives us something with real reference ranges, though they're age-specific. Below are the standard values for women (based on Mayo Clinic clinical ranges):

- 20–29 yrs: 122–436 ng/mL
- 30–39 yrs: 100–370 ng/mL
- 40–49 yrs: 90–310 ng/mL
- 50–59 yrs: 84–240 ng/mL
- 60–69 yrs: 72–225 ng/mL

IGF-1 reflects the brain–body repair economy. Low levels track with poor deep sleep and show up as slow muscle recovery, cognitive dulling, skin aging, and that haunting sentence many women quietly think but rarely say aloud: *No matter what I do, I can't bounce back.* When sleep is chronically fragmented, IGF-1 often follows suit.

### ■ Ghrelin (serum)

There isn't a meaningful universal reference range for ghrelin because it swings with sleep, fasting, stress, time of day, and body composition. Most labs still print ranges, but clinicians treat ghrelin as directional data rather than a target value.

When ghrelin runs high, women usually know it before a lab even confirms it: cravings, carb-hunting at night, emotional hunger, PMS-type mood fluctuations, irritability, and a feeling of "I'm never actually satisfied." Consistently poor sleep drives ghrelin up and nudges hunger cues into overdrive.

## ▨ Leptin (serum)

Leptin does have reference ranges, but they shift with BMI, which means the same number can be "normal" in one woman and clinically significant in another. Most lab ranges for women land between roughly four and twenty-five ng/mL. The more important piece is leptin sensitivity: Lower-end values paired with normal satiety usually reflect metabolic harmony, while higher values are a nudge toward leptin resistance. That's when the brain stops hearing "I'm full" even while the body is broadcasting it. Stress, poor sleep, and the belief that you must "earn" rest push leptin higher, which explains the late-night snacking spiral many women blame on willpower.

## ▨ Beta-Amyloid and Tau Protein (specialty cognitive panels)

These markers don't come with optimal wellness ranges because they aren't used that way. They're diagnostic: Elevated levels or abnormal ratios are used to assess neurodegenerative risk. Their relevance here is simple and sobering. Deep sleep is the time window when the glymphatic system clears amyloid and tau out of the brain. When deep sleep is shortchanged long-term, these proteins accumulate, and the data becomes eerily consistent with future cognitive decline. It's one of the most compelling biological arguments for treating sleep as medicine instead of as a negotiable lifestyle perk.

# PART 6 RECAP:
# DO SOMETHING USELESS

Hobbies and sleep are essential load capacity restoration mechanisms. When you engage in useless, joyful activities, you're actively rebuilding depleted reserves: Flow states increase dopamine and endocannabinoids (mood regulation), creative hobbies boost BDNF (brain repair), and structured play activates your ventral vagal system (safety signaling). Sleep is where the actual restoration happens: Your glymphatic system clears metabolic waste, growth hormone repairs tissues, and memory consolidates. When your Clinical Cues include exhaustion that doesn't improve with rest, creative blocks, emotional flatness, or that "running on fumes" feeling, your load capacity is bottomed out. The labs confirm it: elevated homocysteine, low DHEA-S, disrupted cortisol curves, poor IGF-1. Part 6 gave you permission to do what your nervous system has been begging for: protect rest and play as the biological necessities they are. Your capacity to handle life is directly proportional to how well you protect these restoration practices.

## What We've Learned

**Hobbies are neurological first aid—essential, not optional.** Play is evolutionary. Panksepp and Brown showed that mammals are wired for play the same way we are wired for food and sleep. When you "waste time" on hobbies, you are actually giving your stress system a way to reset instead of staying locked on high alert.

**Flow is your built-in stress vaccination.**

That weirdly timeless zone where you forget to check your phone is a measurable brain state: flow. Flow releases dopamine, norepinephrine, and endocannabinoids in a steady, sustainable pattern. The more often you slip into flow, the faster your brain recovers from stress outside of it.

**Safe play rewires trauma beyond mood regulation.**

Polyvagal theory gave us language for what many trauma clients already knew. Structured, low-stakes play tells your vagus nerve "We are safe now." Painting badly, crocheting crooked scarves, throwing axes at wood instead of people: All of it nudges your body out of survival mode and into connection.

**Hustle culture has been stealing your medicine.**

The minute you turn knitting into a side business or running into a content strategy, the nervous system benefits evaporate. Hobbies only work when they are gloriously useless. Joy that does not have to justify itself is biologically different from joy that is secretly a performance review.

**The "I don't have time" story is a math error.**

You're overinvested in doomscrolling and underinvested in recovery. Time affluence is the feeling of having enough time for what matters. Fifteen minutes of guitar, puzzles, or messy baking moves your brain toward that, even if your calendar does not change.

**Your excuses have a biology, and so does your freedom.**

"I'm not good at anything." "It's indulgent." "I should monetize this." These are stress responses plus cultural conditioning, not logical truths. New skills raise BDNF, CoQ10, vitamin B6 activity, and other repair signals. In other words, your brain literally grows when you let yourself be a beginner.

**Sleep is the night shift for everything you care about.**

Hobbies reclaim your days, but sleep is what rebuilds the hardware. Melatonin, adenosine, GABA, cortisol, serotonin, orexin, and histamine all run the nightclub in your skull. When your rhythms are off, that club turns into chaos. When you protect sleep, those same molecules become your repair crew.

**Your labs quietly confirm the story.**

DHEA-S, homocysteine, lactate, DBH activity, prolactin, leptin, IGF-1, beta-amyloid, and more are biochemical receipts for how much play, rest, and rhythm your system is getting. As hobbies and sleep improve, those markers drift back toward "I can cope with my life" territory.

## Why It Matters

Life is not about to get quieter. Your phone is not going to stop buzzing. The world is not suddenly going to reward you for taking a nap and making lopsided pottery. Waiting for external permission has kept you exhausted, resentful, and convinced that rest is a character flaw instead of a survival skill.

Part 6 gave you a different script. Hobbies = regulation, not extras. Sleep = infrastructure, not treat. Doing something "useless" is how you quietly pull your nervous system out of constant emergency and back into a place where joy, focus, and perspective are even possible.

## Where We Go Next

This is where the science steps back for a minute and something more personal steps in. Before you close the book and go back to everyone else's demands, I want to talk directly to you, human to human, outside of citations and lab ranges.

The next (and final) section is a letter from me to you: not as your scientist friend explaining pathways, but as someone who knows what it's like to live in a brain like ours and still want more than survival.

Read it slowly. Consider it your last permission slip.

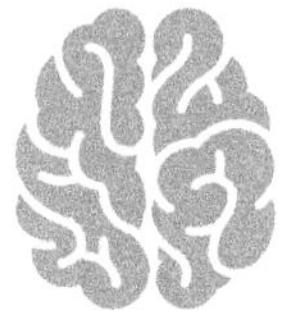



# A LETTER TO YOU

Dear You,

Take a deep breath with me. Slow in, slower out.

There. That right there? That's where the home lives.

If you've made it here, to the very last chapter, I need you to know something. What you've carried, what you've lived through, and the ways you've coped weren't evidence that something was wrong with you.

They were adaptive reflexes from a mind and body doing its best to shield you from overload, fear, hurt, or chaos. The patterns you may have blamed yourself for, like shutting down, bracing, overworking, dissociating, staying on alert, were protection mechanisms. All those ways you felt your body was rebelling or you'd never feel sane? That was your nervous system trying to keep you upright in whatever way it knew.

This book wasn't written to fix you. It was written to help you remember you. To get to know you.

You've traveled through the science of your brain and body, the old wisdom of Stoics and Buddhists, the raw truth about stress, attachment, and burnout. You've collected tools like breath, movement, rest, play. Not as chores, but as your lifelines. You've been given permission to knit badly, dance wildly, nap shamelessly, and practice your peace without apologizing to anyone.

More importantly, you don't have to do all of it. You don't have to get it perfect. You don't even have to remember it all. You just have to choose. One practice, one breath, one moment of awareness at a time. Because again, healing isn't linear; it's circular. It's a beautiful constant. You'll forget and return. Forget and return. And with every return is progress.

I want you to know something else: The way you heal doesn't end with you. When you feel deeply, when you soften, when you laugh, when you sleep, when you play, you send ripples into every nervous system around you. You make others feel safer, calmer, more possible. That is how we change the world. Not through perfection, but through presence.

Your load capacity (your ability to handle stress, regulate emotions, make decisions, and show up for life) is not fixed. It's a dynamic system influenced by everything we've covered: the nutrients feeding your brain, the movement metabolizing your stress, the connections co-regulating your nervous system, the mindfulness creating space in your responses, and the rest restoring your reserves. Every time you check your Clinical Cues and respond to what your body is telling you, you're making a choice to rebuild capacity rather than push through depletion. Some days your capacity will be at 90%, and life will feel manageable. Other days you'll wake up at 20%, and the same tasks will feel impossible. That's biology. The framework helps you recognize where you are and adjust accordingly. When you're depleted, you need more support, simpler tasks, gentler expectations. When you're restored, you have more to give to yourself, to others, to life. This awareness, this skill of reading your own system and responding with compassion rather than judgment, is perhaps the most revolutionary act you can practice.

So if you do nothing else after this, please remember: You are allowed to rest. You are allowed to play. You are allowed to take up space. You are allowed to begin again. Every single day.

Close this book, but don't close the work. Come back to it. Reread the parts that stung or sparked. Share the pieces that made you laugh or cry with someone you love. Let them live beyond these pages because the truth is, your nervous system is not just yours. It's a bridge. It's connection. It's the proof that you were never meant to do this alone.

You already have everything you need inside you. Your body remembers. Your nervous system knows the way home, to homeostasis.

So go ahead. Advocate for yourself, and I'll be cheering you on. Always.

With love and lab data,
Tyla Bee

# LAB TRACKER
## *A Comprehensive Guide to Understanding Your Lab Results*

This lab guide is designed to help you understand what your lab results mean—not just whether they fall within the "normal" reference range, but what they reveal about your overall health and mental wellness. The reference ranges listed are typical values used by most laboratories, but remember: Normal doesn't always mean optimal. The functional ranges represent values associated with optimal function and mental health, not just absence of disease.

*Use this guide alongside your healthcare provider to get a complete picture of your health. Always discuss your results with your doctor before making any changes to your treatment plan.*

# CONTENTS

# 1. Complete Blood Count (CBC)

The CBC measures the cellular components of your blood and is one of the most commonly ordered tests. It provides information about oxygen delivery, immune function, and clotting ability.

### White Blood Cells (WBC)

**What it measures:** The total number of white blood cells, which are your immune system's primary defense against infection and disease.

| Test | Reference Range | Functional Range |
|---|---|---|
| **White Blood Cells (WBC)** | 4.5–11.0 × $10^3$/μL | 5.5–8.0 × $10^3$/μL |

*Mental Health Connection:* Chronic inflammation, indicated by elevated WBC, is strongly linked to depression, anxiety, and brain fog. When your immune system is constantly activated, it produces inflammatory cytokines that can cross the blood–brain barrier and interfere with neurotransmitter function. Low WBC may indicate immune suppression, which can leave you vulnerable to infections that trigger mental health symptoms. Maintaining WBC in the functional range supports both immune resilience and stable mood.

## Red Blood Cells (RBC) — Female

**What it measures:** The number of red blood cells, which carry oxygen from your lungs to every cell in your body.

| Test | Reference Range | Functional Range |
|---|---|---|
| **Red Blood Cells (RBC) — Female** | $4.0–5.5 \times 10^6/\mu L$ | $4.2–4.9 \times 10^6/\mu L$ |

*Mental Health Connection:* Your brain uses about 20% of your body's oxygen despite being only 2% of your body weight. Low RBC count means less oxygen delivery to the brain, which can manifest as fatigue, difficulty concentrating, memory problems, and low mood. Even borderline-low RBC can contribute to that persistent feeling of mental exhaustion that doesn't improve with rest.

## Red Blood Cells (RBC) — Male

**What it measures:** The number of red blood cells, which carry oxygen from your lungs to every cell in your body.

| Test | Reference Range | Functional Range |
|---|---|---|
| **Red Blood Cells (RBC) — Male** | $4.5–6.0 \times 10^6/\mu L$ | $4.7–5.4 \times 10^6/\mu L$ |

*Mental Health Connection:* Your brain requires constant, abundant oxygen to function optimally. Inadequate RBC means insufficient oxygen delivery, leading to cognitive impairment, fatigue, and mood disturbances.

## Hemoglobin (Hgb) - Female

**What it measures:** The protein in red blood cells that actually binds and carries oxygen throughout your body.

| Test | Reference Range | Functional Range |
| --- | --- | --- |
| Hemoglobin (Hgb) — Female | 12.0–16.0 g/dL | 13.5–14.5 g/dL |

***Mental Health Connection:*** Low hemoglobin directly impacts your mental clarity and emotional stability. The brain is extremely sensitive to oxygen levels, and even mild deficiency can cause symptoms that look identical to depression: fatigue, inability to focus, irritability, and lack of motivation. Many women with hemoglobin in the 12–13 g/dL range report significant improvement in mood and energy when they bring levels closer to 14 g/dL.

## Hemoglobin (Hgb) — Male

**What it measures:** The protein in red blood cells that actually binds and carries oxygen throughout your body.

| Test | Reference Range | Functional Range |
| --- | --- | --- |
| Hemoglobin (Hgb) — Male | 14.0–18.0 g/dL | 14.5–15.5 g/dL |

***Mental Health Connection:*** Optimal hemoglobin ensures your brain gets the oxygen it needs for peak cognitive and emotional function. Low levels contribute to brain fog, fatigue, and depressed mood.

## Hematocrit (Hct) — Female

**What it measures:** The percentage of your blood volume made up of red blood cells.

| Test | Reference Range | Functional Range |
| --- | --- | --- |
| Hematocrit (Hct) — Female | 36–46% | 38–42% |

***Mental Health Connection:*** Hematocrit tells a similar story to hemoglobin; it's another measure of your blood's oxygen-carrying capacity. Low hematocrit means your blood is more dilute and less efficient at delivering oxygen to tissues. This can contribute to the physical sensation of anxiety (like not being able to take a deep breath), brain fog, and overwhelming fatigue that makes even simple tasks feel impossible.

## Hematocrit (Hct) — Male

**What it measures:** The percentage of your blood volume made up of red blood cells.

| Test | Reference Range | Functional Range |
| --- | --- | --- |
| Hematocrit (Hct) — Male | 41–53% | 42–48% |

***Mental Health Connection:*** Adequate hematocrit ensures efficient oxygen delivery to all tissues, especially the oxygen-hungry brain. Low levels compromise mental performance and emotional stability.

## Mean Corpuscular Volume (MCV)

**What it measures:** The average size of your red blood cells.

| Test | Reference Range | Functional Range |
| --- | --- | --- |
| Mean Corpuscular Volume (MCV) | 80–100 fL | 85–92 fL |

*Mental Health Connection:* MCV helps identify the cause of anemia. Low MCV (microcytic) typically indicates iron deficiency, which is extremely common in menstruating women and directly impacts neurotransmitter production. High MCV (macrocytic) can indicate B12 or folate deficiency, both critical for methylation, the process that regulates neurotransmitters like serotonin and dopamine. If your MCV is outside the optimal range, it's a clue about which nutrients you need to support brain function.

## Mean Corpuscular Hemoglobin (MCH)

**What it measures:** The average amount of hemoglobin in each red blood cell.

| Test | Reference Range | Functional Range |
| --- | --- | --- |
| Mean Corpuscular Hemoglobin (MCH) | 27–33 pg | 28–31 pg |

*Mental Health Connection:* MCH correlates with MCV and helps confirm nutrient deficiencies. Low MCH typically accompanies iron deficiency, while high MCH suggests vitamin B deficiency. Both scenarios compromise your brain's ability to produce adequate neurotransmitters and maintain stable energy levels throughout the day.

## Mean Corpuscular Hemoglobin Concentration (MCHC)

**What it measures:** The concentration of hemoglobin in a given volume of red blood cells.

| Test | Reference Range | Functional Range |
| --- | --- | --- |
| Mean Corpuscular Hemoglobin Concentration (MCHC) | 32–36 g/dL | 33–35 g/dL |

*Mental Health Connection:* MCHC is one of the most stable red blood cell indices and changes slowly. Abnormal MCHC can indicate chronic conditions affecting red blood cell production. While it's less directly tied to acute mental health symptoms, chronic low MCHC contributes to persistent fatigue and cognitive dysfunction.

## Red Cell Distribution Width (RDW)

**What it measures:** The variation in size of your red blood cells (how much they differ from each other).

| Test | Reference Range | Functional Range |
| --- | --- | --- |
| Red Cell Distribution Width (RDW) | 11.5–14.5% | 11.5–13.5% |

*Mental Health Connection:* Elevated RDW indicates your body is producing red blood cells of varying sizes, which often happens during nutritional deficiency recovery or chronic inflammation. High RDW has been associated with increased inflammation and oxidative stress, both of which impair brain function and contribute to depression and anxiety. It's also an early marker that something is affecting your red blood cell production before you become overtly anemic.

## Platelets

**What it measures:** The number of platelets, which are cell fragments responsible for blood clotting.

| Test | Reference Range | Functional Range |
| --- | --- | --- |
| **Platelets** | 150–400 × $10^3$/μL | 175–250 × $10^3$/μL |

***Mental Health Connection:*** While platelets are primarily known for clotting, they also store and release serotonin. In fact, about 95% of your body's serotonin is found in platelets and the gut, not in the brain. Platelet dysfunction or abnormal counts can affect serotonin regulation throughout the body. Additionally, elevated platelets can indicate chronic inflammation, which impacts mood and cognitive function.

# 2. Comprehensive Metabolic Panel (CMP)

The CMP measures how well your kidneys and liver are working, your blood sugar levels, and your body's electrolyte and acid-base balance. These tests provide a window into your metabolic health.

### Fasting Glucose

**What it measures:** The amount of sugar (glucose) in your blood, which is your body's primary fuel source.

| Test | Reference Range | Functional Range |
|---|---|---|
| **Fasting Glucose** | 70–99 mg/dL | 75–85 mg/dL |

***Mental Health Connection:*** Your brain requires a constant, stable supply of glucose to function. Blood sugar dysregulation—whether too high or too low—has profound effects on mood, anxiety, and cognitive function. Low blood sugar triggers the release of stress hormones like cortisol and adrenaline, which can cause irritability, shakiness, anxiety, and difficulty concentrating. High blood sugar, especially chronically elevated levels, damages blood vessels throughout the body, including in the brain, contributing to inflammation and increasing risk for depression. Many people with blood sugar in the 90–99 mg/dL range feel significantly better when they bring it into the 75–85 mg/dL range through dietary changes.

### Hemoglobin A1c (HbA1c)

**What it measures:** The average blood sugar level over the past two-to-three months by measuring the percentage of hemoglobin coated with sugar.

| Test | Reference Range | Functional Range |
|---|---|---|
| Hemoglobin A1c (HbA1c) | <5.7% | 4.8–5.2% |

***Mental Health Connection:*** Hemoglobin A1c shows your long-term blood sugar control, which has profound effects on brain health and mood. Elevated A1c (even in the pre-diabetic range of 5.7–6.4%) indicates chronic blood sugar dysregulation that damages blood vessels throughout the body, including in the brain. This damage contributes to inflammation, oxidative stress, and impaired neurotransmitter function. High A1c is associated with increased risk of depression, anxiety, cognitive decline, and dementia. Blood sugar fluctuations cause energy crashes, irritability, brain fog, and difficulty concentrating. Many people with A1c in the 5.5–5.7% range (considered "normal") experience significant improvements in mood stability, energy, and mental clarity when they bring it below 5.3% through dietary changes. Chronically elevated blood sugar also impairs the blood–brain barrier, allowing inflammatory molecules to enter the brain more easily.

## Blood Urea Nitrogen (BUN)

**What it measures:** Urea nitrogen in your blood, a waste product from protein breakdown that your kidneys filter out.

| Test | Reference Range | Functional Range |
|---|---|---|
| Blood Urea Nitrogen (BUN) | 7–20 mg/dL | 10–16 mg/dL |

***Mental Health Connection:*** BUN reflects both kidney function and protein metabolism. Very low BUN can indicate inadequate protein intake, which means you're not getting enough amino acids to make neurotransmitters like serotonin, dopamine, and GABA. High BUN can indicate dehydration, which impairs cognitive function and mood, or kidney dysfunction, which allows toxins to build up in your system and affect mental clarity.

## Creatinine — Female

**What it measures:** A waste product from normal muscle breakdown that kidneys filter from your blood.

| Test | Reference Range | Functional Range |
|---|---|---|
| **Creatinine — Female** | 0.6–1.2 mg/dL | 0.7–1.0 mg/dL |

***Mental Health Connection:*** Creatinine is primarily a marker of kidney function. When kidneys aren't filtering properly, waste products and toxins accumulate in the bloodstream, which can cause cognitive impairment, confusion, fatigue, and mood changes. Very low creatinine can indicate low muscle mass, which often accompanies chronic stress, inadequate nutrition, or conditions that affect mental health.

## Creatinine — Male

**What it measures:** A waste product from normal muscle breakdown that kidneys filter from your blood.

| Test | Reference Range | Functional Range |
|---|---|---|
| **Creatinine — Male** | 0.7–1.3 mg/dL | 0.8–1.1 mg/dL |

***Mental Health Connection:*** Adequate kidney function is essential for clearing metabolic waste that can impair brain function. Low creatinine may reflect poor muscle mass or chronic illness affecting overall health.

## eGFR

**What it measures:** How well your kidneys are filtering waste from your blood, calculated from your creatinine level, age, and sex.

| Test | Reference Range | Functional Range |
|---|---|---|
| **eGFR** | >60 mL/min/1.73m$^2$ | >90 mL/min/1.73m$^2$ |

***Mental Health Connection:*** eGFR gives a more complete picture of kidney function than creatinine alone. Declining kidney function means your body is less efficient at clearing metabolic waste, medications, and toxins. This can lead to uremia, a condition where waste products build up in the blood and cause significant cognitive and mood changes, including confusion, difficulty concentrating, and depression.

## Sodium (Na)

**What it measures:** The main electrolyte in your extracellular fluid, critical for nerve and muscle function.

| Test | Reference Range | Functional Range |
|---|---|---|
| **Sodium (Na)** | 136–145 mEq/L | 138–142 mEq/L |

***Mental Health Connection:*** Sodium is essential for nerve signal transmission, including in the brain. Both low sodium (hyponatremia) and high sodium (hypernatremia) can cause neurological symptoms. Low sodium can cause confusion, headaches, irritability, fatigue, and in severe cases, seizures. Even mild chronic low sodium can contribute to cognitive impairment and mood changes. High sodium is less common but can cause confusion, lethargy, and in severe cases, altered consciousness.

## Potassium (K)

**What it measures:** An essential electrolyte for heart, nerve, and muscle function.

| Test | Reference Range | Functional Range |
|---|---|---|
| **Potassium (K)** | 3.5–5.0 mEq/L | 4.0–4.5 mEq/L |

***Mental Health Connection:*** Potassium is crucial for proper nerve function. Low potassium can cause weakness, fatigue, muscle cramps, and in the brain, can contribute to confusion and mood changes. Potassium works in tandem with sodium to generate the electrical signals that neurons use to communicate. Imbalances can disrupt this signaling, leading to cognitive dysfunction. Additionally, low potassium is associated with increased anxiety and stress response.

## Chloride (Cl)

**What it measures:** An electrolyte that helps maintain proper fluid balance and acid-base balance in your body.

| Test | Reference Range | Functional Range |
|---|---|---|
| **Chloride (Cl)** | 98–107 mEq/L | 100–106 mEq/L |

***Mental Health Connection:*** Chloride helps produce stomach acid for digestion and works with sodium to maintain fluid balance. Abnormal chloride levels usually indicate acid-base imbalances in the body. While less directly tied to mental health than other electrolytes, severe imbalances can cause confusion, weakness, and difficulty breathing, which certainly affects mental state and anxiety levels.

## Carbon Dioxide (CO2)

**What it measures:** The amount of bicarbonate ($HCO_3^-$) in your blood, which helps maintain your body's pH balance.

| Test | Reference Range | Functional Range |
|---|---|---|
| **Carbon Dioxide (CO2)** | 23–29 mEq/L | 25–28 mEq/L |

***Mental Health Connection:*** CO2 (measured as bicarbonate) reflects your body's acid-base balance. Low CO2 can indicate metabolic acidosis, which can cause confusion, fatigue, rapid breathing, and headaches. High CO2 can indicate respiratory issues or metabolic alkalosis, which can cause confusion, muscle twitching, and lethargy. The brain is extremely sensitive to pH changes, and even subtle acid-base imbalances can affect cognitive function and mood.

## Calcium (Ca)

**What it measures:** The level of calcium in your blood, essential for bone health, muscle contraction, nerve signaling, and blood clotting.

| Test | Reference Range | Functional Range |
| --- | --- | --- |
| Calcium (Ca) | 8.5–10.5 mg/dL | 9.0–10.0 mg/dL |

***Mental Health Connection:*** Calcium is critical for nerve signal transmission and neurotransmitter release. Low calcium can cause anxiety, irritability, depression, confusion, and memory problems. It also plays a role in the stress response; calcium is necessary for cortisol production, and imbalances can dysregulate your stress system. High calcium can cause fatigue, depression, difficulty concentrating, and in severe cases, confusion and altered mental status.

## Total Protein

**What it measures:** The combined amount of albumin and globulins in your blood.

| Test | Reference Range | Functional Range |
| --- | --- | --- |
| Total Protein | 6.0–8.3 g/dL | 6.9–7.4 g/dL |

***Mental Health Connection:*** Total protein reflects your overall protein status. Low protein can indicate malnutrition or malabsorption, which means you're not getting the amino acids needed to build neurotransmitters. Every neurotransmitter—serotonin, dopamine, GABA, norepinephrine—is made from amino acids derived from dietary protein. Chronically low protein contributes to depression, anxiety, poor concentration, and lack of motivation.

## Albumin

**What it measures:** The most abundant protein in your blood, made by your liver, which helps maintain fluid balance and transports hormones, vitamins, and medications.

| Test | Reference Range | Functional Range |
|---|---|---|
| **Albumin** | 3.5–5.5 g/dL | 4.0–4.8 g/dL |

*Mental Health Connection:* Albumin is essential for transporting thyroid hormones, sex hormones, and cortisol throughout your body. Low albumin can lead to inadequate hormone delivery to the brain, affecting mood, energy, and cognitive function. It's also a marker of chronic inflammation and oxidative stress conditions that are strongly linked to depression and anxiety. Albumin levels in the lower end of the reference range often indicate chronic stress or inadequate protein intake.

## Globulin

**What it measures:** A group of proteins including antibodies and transport proteins, calculated as total protein minus albumin.

| Test | Reference Range | Functional Range |
|---|---|---|
| **Globulin** | 2.0–3.5 g/dL | 2.3–2.8 g/dL |

*Mental Health Connection:* Globulins include your antibodies (immunoglobulins), so elevated levels often indicate chronic immune activation or infection. Chronic inflammation from an overactive immune system is one of the strongest biological contributors to depression and anxiety. The inflammatory cytokines produced during immune responses can cross into the brain and directly affect mood, motivation, and cognitive function.

## A/G Ratio

**What it measures:** The ratio of albumin to globulin, calculated by dividing albumin by globulin.

| Test | Reference Range | Functional Range |
| --- | --- | --- |
| A/G Ratio | 1.0-2.5 | 1.5–2.2 |

***Mental Health Connection:*** The A/G ratio is a quick indicator of the balance between inflammation and nutritional status. A low ratio (high globulin relative to albumin) suggests chronic inflammation or immune activation, both of which are strongly linked to depression and cognitive dysfunction. A high ratio might indicate inadequate immune function or dehydration.

## Alkaline Phosphatase (ALP)

**What it measures:** An enzyme found in your liver, bones, and other tissues that helps break down proteins.

| Test | Reference Range | Functional Range |
| --- | --- | --- |
| Alkaline Phosphatase (ALP) | 44–147 U/L | 50–100 U/L |

***Mental Health Connection:*** ALP is primarily a marker of liver and bone health. Elevated ALP can indicate liver dysfunction or vitamin D deficiency (the body increases ALP to try to compensate for poor bone mineralization). Both liver problems and vitamin D deficiency are associated with depression, fatigue, and cognitive impairment. The liver is crucial for detoxification and hormone metabolism, so dysfunction here can lead to a buildup of substances that affect brain function.

## Alanine Aminotransferase (ALT)

**What it measures:** An enzyme found primarily in the liver; elevated levels indicate liver cell damage.

| Test | Reference Range | Functional Range |
| --- | --- | --- |
| **Alanine Aminotransferase (ALT)** | 7–56 U/L | 10–26 U/L |

***Mental Health Connection:*** ALT is a sensitive marker of liver inflammation and damage. Your liver is responsible for detoxifying everything you're exposed to and metabolizing hormones. When liver function is compromised, toxins accumulate and hormones become imbalanced, both of which affect brain function. Many people with chronically elevated ALT (even within the reference range) report improved mood, energy, and mental clarity when they address the underlying causes of liver inflammation through diet and lifestyle changes.

## Aspartate Aminotransferase (AST)

**What it measures:** An enzyme found in the liver, heart, muscles, and other tissues. Elevated levels can indicate damage to these tissues.

| Test | Reference Range | Functional Range |
| --- | --- | --- |
| Aspartate Aminotransferase (AST) | 10–40 U/L | 15–30 U/L |

*Mental Health Connection:* AST is found in many tissues, so elevation can indicate various forms of cellular damage. The AST-to-ALT ratio helps determine if liver damage is present (ratio typically elevated in liver disease). Like ALT, elevated AST indicates cellular inflammation and dysfunction, which impairs detoxification and hormone metabolism, both critical for mental health.

## Total Bilirubin

**What it measures:** A yellow pigment produced during the normal breakdown of red blood cells. Processed by the liver.

| Test | Reference Range | Functional Range |
| --- | --- | --- |
| **Total Bilirubin** | 0.1–1.2 mg/dL | 0.2–0.9 mg/dL |

*Mental Health Connection:* Bilirubin reflects how well your liver is processing waste products from red blood cell breakdown. Elevated bilirubin can indicate liver dysfunction, which impairs detoxification and leads to accumulation of substances that affect brain function. Interestingly, mildly elevated bilirubin (within the reference range) can sometimes be protective due to its antioxidant properties, but significantly elevated levels indicate problems that need attention.

# 3. Iron Panel

The iron panel measures how much iron your body has and how well it's being transported and stored. Iron is essential for oxygen delivery and energy production, making it critical for mental health.

### Serum Iron — Female

**What it measures:** The amount of iron circulating in your blood at the time of the test.

| Test | Reference Range | Functional Range |
| --- | --- | --- |
| Serum Iron — Female | 50–170 µg/dL | 85–130 µg/dL |

***Mental Health Connection:*** Serum iron fluctuates throughout the day and with meals, so it's best interpreted alongside ferritin and TIBC. Low serum iron contributes to fatigue, weakness, and poor concentration, but this marker alone doesn't tell the full story. It's part of the bigger picture of iron status.

### Serum Iron — Male

**What it measures:** The amount of iron circulating in your blood at the time of the test.

| Test | Reference Range | Functional Range |
| --- | --- | --- |
| Serum Iron — Male | 65–175 µg/dL | 95–150 µg/dL |

***Mental Health Connection:*** While serum iron provides a snapshot, it must be considered with other iron markers for a complete assessment of iron status and its impact on energy and cognition.

## Ferritin — Female

**What it measures:** Your body's iron storage protein, giving the best indication of total body iron stores.

| Test | Reference Range | Functional Range |
| --- | --- | --- |
| Ferritin — Female | 12–150 ng/mL | 50–100 ng/mL |

***Mental Health Connection:*** Ferritin is arguably the most important marker for mental health in the iron panel. Iron is required for the production of neurotransmitters, including serotonin, dopamine, and norepinephrine. It's also essential for myelin formation (the insulation around nerve fibers) and energy production in brain cells. Low ferritin—even when hemoglobin is normal—is strongly associated with depression, anxiety, brain fog, poor concentration, and fatigue. Many women with ferritin levels in the 12–30 ng/mL range (technically "normal") experience dramatic improvements in mood, energy, and cognitive function when they bring levels up to 80–100 ng/mL. Note that ferritin is also an acute phase reactant, meaning it can be falsely elevated during inflammation or infection.

## Ferritin — Male

**What it measures:** Your body's iron storage protein, giving the best indication of total body iron stores.

| Test | Reference Range | Functional Range |
| --- | --- | --- |
| Ferritin — Male | 12–300 ng/mL | 75–150 ng/mL |

*Mental Health Connection:* Adequate ferritin stores are essential for optimal brain function, neurotransmitter synthesis, and sustained energy. Low levels impair mental performance even before anemia develops.

## Total Iron Binding Capacity (TIBC)

**What it measures:** The maximum amount of iron your blood can carry, which reflects the amount of transferrin (the protein that transports iron).

| Test | Reference Range | Functional Range |
| --- | --- | --- |
| Total Iron Binding Capacity (TIBC) | 250–450 µg/dL | 300–380 µg/dL |

*Mental Health Connection:* TIBC tends to increase when iron stores are low (the body makes more transferrin to try to capture more iron) and decrease when iron stores are adequate. When TIBC is high, it suggests your body is desperately trying to find and transport more iron. This pattern, combined with low ferritin, indicates iron deficiency that's likely affecting your energy, mood, and cognitive function.

## Transferrin Saturation (TSAT)

**What it measures:** The percentage of transferrin (iron transport protein) that's actually carrying iron, calculated as (serum iron ÷ TIBC) × 100.

| Test | Reference Range | Functional Range |
| --- | --- | --- |
| Transferrin Saturation (TSAT) | 20–50% | 25–35% |

***Mental Health Connection:*** Transferrin saturation shows how efficiently iron is being transported in your blood. Low TSAT (under 20%) indicates iron deficiency and means your tissues—including your brain—aren't getting enough iron for optimal function. This directly impacts neurotransmitter production, energy levels, and cognitive performance. Many people with TSAT in the teens report significant improvements in mental clarity and mood when they bring it above 25%.

# 4. Special Chemistry

Special chemistry tests measure vitamins, minerals, inflammatory markers, and other substances that have significant impacts on mental health and well-being.

### Vitamin D (25-hydroxyvitamin D)

**What it measures:** The level of vitamin D in your blood, which functions as both a vitamin and a hormone.

| Test | Reference Range | Functional Range |
|---|---|---|
| Vitamin D (25-hydroxyvitamin D) | 30–100 ng/mL | 50–70 ng/mL |

*Mental Health Connection:* Vitamin D is crucial for brain health and has receptors throughout the nervous system. Low vitamin D is strongly associated with depression, anxiety, seasonal affective disorder, and cognitive decline. Vitamin D regulates the production of neurotransmitters, modulates inflammation in the brain, and protects neurons from damage. Many people with levels in the 30–40 ng/mL range (considered "sufficient" by medical standards) report significant mood improvements when they bring levels up to 60–70 ng/mL. Vitamin D deficiency is extremely common, especially in those living far from the equator or with limited sun exposure.

### Vitamin B12 (Cobalamin)

**What it measures:** The level of vitamin B12 in your blood, essential for nerve function and red blood cell production.

| Test | Reference Range | Functional Range |
| --- | --- | --- |
| **Vitamin B12 (Cobalamin)** | 200–900 pg/mL | 500–800 pg/mL |

***Mental Health Connection:*** B12 is absolutely critical for mental health. It's required for myelin production (the protective coating around nerves), neurotransmitter synthesis, and methylation—a biochemical process that regulates mood and detoxification. B12 deficiency can cause symptoms identical to depression, including fatigue, difficulty concentrating, memory problems, irritability, and mood changes. It can also cause neurological symptoms like tingling, numbness, and balance problems. Many people with B12 levels in the 200–400 pg/mL range experience significant improvements in energy, mood, and cognitive clarity when they bring levels above 500 pg/mL. B12 deficiency is common in vegans, vegetarians, people over fifty, and those with digestive issues.

## Folate (Folic Acid)

**What it measures:** The level of folate in your blood, a B vitamin essential for DNA synthesis and methylation.

| Test | Reference Range | Functional Range |
| --- | --- | --- |
| **Folate (Folic Acid)** | >3.0 ng/mL | 10–20 ng/mL |

***Mental Health Connection:*** Folate works hand in hand with B12 in methylation pathways that are critical for neurotransmitter production and regulation. Low folate is associated with depression, anxiety, cognitive decline, and poor response to antidepressant medications. Some people have genetic variations (like MTHFR polymorphisms) that impair their ability to convert folic acid to its active form, methylfolate. For these individuals, even "normal" folate levels may not translate to adequate brain function, and supplementation with methylfolate can be life-changing.

## Methylmalonic Acid (MMA)

**What it measures:** A metabolic byproduct that accumulates when your body doesn't have enough functional B12 to complete a critical enzymatic reaction. It's considered the most sensitive and specific marker of true B12 deficiency at the cellular level.

| Test | Reference Range | Functional Range |
| --- | --- | --- |
| **Methylmalonic Acid (MMA)** | <0.4 μmol/L | <0.27 μmol/L |

*Mental Health Connection:* MMA is the lab that catches the B12 deficiency your serum B12 missed. A woman can have a serum B12 of 350 pg/mL (well within "normal") and still have elevated MMA, meaning her cells are functionally starving for B12. This matters because B12 is essential for myelin production (nerve insulation), neurotransmitter synthesis, methylation, and energy metabolism in the brain. Elevated MMA is associated with fatigue, brain fog, numbness and tingling, depression, anxiety, and memory problems. It's especially important for women who are plant-based, on metformin, on oral contraceptives, or who have gut issues that impair absorption

(Crohn's, celiac, SIBO, chronic PPI use). If your B12 looks "fine" but you still feel like a zombie, MMA is the test that tells the truth. Think of serum B12 as checking whether the groceries were delivered. MMA tells you whether anyone actually cooked dinner.

### Magnesium (Serum)

**What it measures:** The level of magnesium in your blood, a mineral involved in over 300 biochemical reactions.

| Test | Reference Range | Functional Range |
| --- | --- | --- |
| **Magnesium (Serum)** | 1.7–2.2 mg/dL | 2.0–2.2 mg/dL |

***Mental Health Connection:*** Magnesium is often called the "relaxation mineral" because it helps regulate the nervous system and stress response. It's essential for GABA function (your calming neurotransmitter), energy production, and hundreds of other processes. Low magnesium is associated with anxiety, depression, insomnia, muscle tension, and headaches. However, serum magnesium is a poor indicator of total body magnesium status because only 1% of your body's magnesium is in the blood; most is stored in bones and tissues. Many people have inadequate magnesium despite normal blood levels. Red blood cell (RBC) magnesium is a better test if available, but many people benefit from magnesium supplementation even with "normal" serum levels, especially if they have symptoms of deficiency.

## RBC Magnesium (Red Blood Cell Magnesium)

**What it measures:** The amount of magnesium inside your red blood cells, reflecting your body's true intracellular magnesium stores rather than the small fraction circulating in blood.

| Test | Reference Range | Functional Range |
|---|---|---|
| **RBC Magnesium** | 4.2-6.8 mg/dL | 5.5-6.5 mg/dL |

*Mental Health Connection:* This is the magnesium test your provider probably isn't running, and it's the one that actually matters. Serum magnesium (the standard test) only measures the 1% of your total magnesium floating in the blood. Your body will pull magnesium from cells and bones to keep serum levels stable. RBC magnesium reflects what's available inside your cells, where magnesium does its work: activating GABA receptors, regulating the stress response, supporting serotonin production, and calming neural excitability. Low RBC magnesium is associated with anxiety, insomnia, PMS, migraines, muscle tension, and heightened stress reactivity. Women on oral contraceptives, women under chronic stress, and women who drink alcohol regularly are at highest risk for intracellular depletion. If your serum magnesium is "normal" but you're anxious, can't sleep, and cramp before your period, request the RBC test. It's the difference between checking the gas gauge on the dashboard and actually looking in the tank.

## Homocysteine

**What it measures:** An amino acid in your blood. Elevated levels indicate problems with methylation and B vitamin status.

| Test | Reference Range | Functional Range |
| --- | --- | --- |
| **Homocysteine** | 5–15 μmol/L | 6–9 μmol/L |

***Mental Health Connection:*** Homocysteine is a marker of methylation efficiency and B vitamin status (especially B12, folate, and B6). Elevated homocysteine indicates impaired methylation, which is critical for neurotransmitter production and regulation. High homocysteine is associated with depression, cognitive decline, and increased risk of dementia and cardiovascular disease. It also indicates inflammation and oxidative stress, both of which impair brain function. Many people with homocysteine in the 10–15 μmol/L range (technically "normal") feel significantly better when they bring it below 9 through B vitamin supplementation.

## High-Sensitivity C-Reactive Protein (hs-CRP)

**What it measures:** A marker of inflammation in your body.

| Test | Reference Range | Functional Range |
| --- | --- | --- |
| **High-Sensitivity C-Reactive Protein (hs-CRP)** | <3.0 mg/L | <1.0 mg/L |

***Mental Health Connection:*** hs-CRP is one of the most important markers for mental health because it measures systemic inflammation. Elevated CRP is strongly associated with depression, anxiety, and cognitive dysfunction. Inflammation interferes with neurotransmitter production, damages brain cells, and disrupts the blood–brain barrier.

Even mildly elevated CRP (in the 1–3 mg/L range) can contribute to mood problems and brain fog. Ideally, CRP should be well below 1.0 mg/L for optimal mental health. Chronic inflammation is one of the most significant modifiable risk factors for depression.

### Fasting Insulin

**What it measures:** The amount of insulin in your blood after an overnight fast, reflecting how hard your pancreas is working to keep blood sugar stable.

| Test | Reference Range | Functional Range |
| --- | --- | --- |
| **Fasting Insulin** | 2–25 µIU/mL | 2–5 µIU/mL |

***Mental Health Connection:*** Fasting insulin is one of the most important—and most overlooked—markers for mental health. Elevated fasting insulin (>10 µIU/mL) indicates insulin resistance, even when blood sugar and A1c are still "normal." Insulin resistance means your cells aren't responding efficiently to insulin, so your pancreas produces more to compensate. This creates a cascade of problems for the brain: chronic inflammation, impaired glucose delivery to brain cells, disrupted neurotransmitter function, and hormonal imbalances.

High insulin is strongly associated with depression, anxiety, brain fog, and increased dementia risk. It also contributes to PCOS, which has high rates of depression and anxiety. Many people with insulin levels in the 10–15 µIU/mL range (technically "normal") are already experiencing insulin resistance and its mental health consequences. Bringing insulin below 5 µIU/mL through dietary changes (especially reducing refined carbohydrates and increasing protein/fat) often results in dramatic improvements in mood, energy, and cognitive function. This is one of the earliest markers of metabolic dysfunction; it rises years before glucose becomes abnormal.

## Omega-3 Index

**What it measures:** The percentage of EPA and DHA (omega-3 fatty acids) in red blood cell membranes, reflecting your tissue levels of these essential fats.

| Test | Reference Range | Functional Range |
| --- | --- | --- |
| **Omega-3 Index** | N/A | >8% |

***Mental Health Connection:*** Omega-3 fatty acids, particularly EPA and DHA, are critical structural components of brain cell membranes and are essential for neurotransmitter function, neuroplasticity, and reducing brain inflammation. Low omega-3 levels (<4%) are strongly associated with depression, anxiety, cognitive decline, and increased suicide risk. The Omega-3 Index is one of the most modifiable risk factors for mental health. Supplementation with high-quality fish oil can significantly improve this marker within three-to-four months. Studies show that omega-3 supplementation can be as effective as antidepressants for some people with depression, particularly when their baseline levels are low. An Omega-3 Index below 8% suggests your brain doesn't have the building blocks it needs for optimal function. This is especially important for anyone with a history of depression, anxiety, or cognitive issues, and for anyone who doesn't regularly eat fatty fish.

## Zinc (Serum)

**What it measures:** The level of zinc in your blood. RBC (red blood cell) zinc is a better measure of tissue stores than serum zinc.

| Test | Reference Range | Functional Range |
|---|---|---|
| **Zinc (Serum)** | 60–120 µg/dL | 90–110 µg/dL |

***Mental Health Connection:*** Zinc is essential for neurotransmitter function, immune regulation, and antioxidant protection in the brain. It's required for the synthesis and signaling of serotonin, dopamine, and GABA. Zinc deficiency is extremely common, especially in people with digestive issues, vegetarians/vegans, and those under chronic stress. Low zinc is associated with depression, anxiety, ADHD, poor memory, and increased inflammation. Zinc also modulates the stress response and helps regulate the HPA (hypothalamic-pituitary-adrenal) axis. Many antidepressants work better when zinc levels are adequate. Even mild zinc deficiency can impair taste and smell, contribute to poor appetite, and worsen mood. Serum zinc is not a great marker, because it doesn't reflect tissue stores well; if you can get RBC zinc tested, that's more accurate. Supplementation (25–50 mg daily) often improves mood and cognitive function in people with low levels, though it's important not to overdo it as excess zinc can interfere with copper absorption.

## GGT (Gamma-Glutamyl Transferase)

**What it measures:** An enzyme found primarily in the liver. Elevated levels indicate liver stress, even when other liver enzymes are normal.

| Test | Reference Range | Functional Range |
| --- | --- | --- |
| GGT (Gamma-Glutamyl Transferase) | 9–38 U/L | <20 U/L |

***Mental Health Connection:*** GGT is a more sensitive marker of liver dysfunction and oxidative stress than ALT or AST. It rises with alcohol consumption, fatty liver disease, medication use, and environmental toxin exposure. Elevated GGT indicates your liver is under stress and struggling with detoxification, which allows toxins and inflammatory molecules to circulate and affect brain function. High GGT (>40 U/L) is associated with increased inflammation, insulin resistance, and cognitive decline. Even GGT in the 25–40 U/L range (technically "normal") suggests room for improvement in liver health and detoxification capacity, which can impact mood and mental clarity.

## ESR (Erythrocyte Sedimentation Rate)

**What it measures:** How quickly red blood cells settle in a test tube. Faster settling indicates inflammation.

| Test | Reference Range | Functional Range |
| --- | --- | --- |
| ESR (Erythrocyte Sedimentation Rate) | 0–20 mm/hr | <10 mm/hr |

***Mental Health Connection:*** ESR is a nonspecific marker of inflammation; it rises with infections, autoimmune diseases, and chronic inflammation. Like CRP, elevated ESR indicates systemic inflammation that can affect brain function. ESR >20 mm/hr suggests active inflammation that warrants investigation. While less sensitive than hs-CRP, ESR can pick up different types of inflammation (especially related to autoimmune conditions) and is useful as a complementary marker.

# 5. Lipid Panel

The lipid panel measures fats (lipids) in your blood. While primarily used to assess cardiovascular risk, these markers have significant implications for brain health. Your brain is 60% fat, and cholesterol is essential for myelin formation, neurotransmitter function, and cell membrane integrity.

### Total Cholesterol

**What it measures:** The total amount of cholesterol in your blood, including both "good" HDL and "bad" LDL cholesterol.

| Test | Reference Range | Functional Range |
| --- | --- | --- |
| **Total Cholesterol** | <200 mg/dL | 160–220 mg/dL |

***Mental Health Connection:*** Cholesterol has a complex relationship with mental health. While very high cholesterol (>240 mg/dL) is associated with cardiovascular disease and cognitive decline, cholesterol that's too low (<160 mg/dL) is also problematic for brain function. Cholesterol is essential for making steroid hormones, vitamin D, and maintaining cell membranes—all critical for brain health. Studies show that very low cholesterol is associated with increased depression, anxiety, and even suicidal ideation. Your brain needs adequate cholesterol to function. The key is finding the sweet spot: not too high, not too low.

## LDL Cholesterol

**What it measures:** The "bad" cholesterol that can build up in artery walls; however, LDL is also essential for transporting cholesterol to tissues that need it, including the brain.

| Test | Reference Range | Functional Range |
|---|---|---|
| **LDL Cholesterol** | <100 mg/dL | 80–120 mg/dL |

*Mental Health Connection:* LDL's relationship with mental health is nuanced. While very high LDL contributes to vascular damage that impairs brain function, excessively low LDL (<70 mg/dL) has been associated with increased depression and mood instability. LDL particles carry cholesterol to your brain cells, which need it for neurotransmitter receptor function and cell membrane integrity. The quality of LDL particles matters more than the number; small, dense LDL particles are more inflammatory and damaging, while large, fluffy LDL particles are less concerning. If your LDL is very low and you're experiencing depression or mood issues, it's worth discussing with your doctor.

## HDL Cholesterol

**What it measures:** The "good" cholesterol that helps remove excess cholesterol from your bloodstream and has anti-inflammatory properties.

| Test | Reference Range | Functional Range |
|---|---|---|
| **HDL Cholesterol** | >40 mg/dL (men), >50 mg/dL (women) | >60 mg/dL |

***Mental Health Connection:*** HDL is protective for both cardiovascular and brain health. Higher HDL is associated with better cognitive function, lower inflammation, and reduced risk of depression. HDL has antioxidant and anti-inflammatory properties that protect the brain from damage. Low HDL (<40 mg/dL) is often seen alongside metabolic dysfunction, chronic inflammation, and insulin resistance—all of which impair brain function and contribute to depression and anxiety. Exercise and omega-3 fatty acids are among the most effective ways to raise HDL naturally.

## Triglycerides

**What it measures:** The amount of fat (triglycerides) circulating in your blood, which reflects how your body processes dietary fats and carbohydrates.

| Test | Reference Range | Functional Range |
|---|---|---|
| **Triglycerides** | <150 mg/dL | <100 mg/dL |

***Mental Health Connection:*** Elevated triglycerides indicate metabolic dysfunction and are strongly associated with insulin resistance, inflammation, and poor brain health. High triglycerides (>150 mg/dL) are linked to increased depression, anxiety, cognitive impairment, and increased risk of dementia. Triglycerides compete with essential nutrients for transport across the blood–brain barrier, potentially limiting the brain's access to important compounds. They're also a marker of blood sugar dysregulation; high-carbohydrate diets and frequent eating spike triglycerides. Many people with triglycerides in the

120–150 mg/dL range (technically "normal") see dramatic improvements in mental clarity, mood, and energy when they bring levels below 100 mg/dL through dietary changes, particularly reducing refined carbohydrates and increasing omega-3 fatty acids.

## Cholesterol-to-HDL Ratio

**What it measures:** Total cholesterol divided by HDL cholesterol. This ratio is often a better predictor of cardiovascular risk than total cholesterol alone.

| Test | Reference Range | Functional Range |
|---|---|---|
| Cholesterol-to-HDL Ratio | <5.0 | <3.5 |

*Mental Health Connection:* The cholesterol-to-HDL ratio reflects the balance between potentially harmful and protective cholesterol. A high ratio (>5.0) indicates higher inflammation and metabolic dysfunction, both of which impair brain function. This ratio is associated with insulin resistance, chronic inflammation, and increased risk of depression and cognitive decline. A ratio above 4.0, even with "normal" individual values, suggests room for improvement in metabolic health that could benefit mental wellness.

# 6. Immunology

Immunology tests assess your immune system function and can identify autoimmune conditions and thyroid disorders that significantly impact mental health.

### Thyroid Stimulating Hormone (TSH)

**What it measures:** A hormone produced by your pituitary gland that signals your thyroid to produce thyroid hormones.

| Test | Reference Range | Functional Range |
| --- | --- | --- |
| **Thyroid Stimulating Hormone (TSH)** | 0.4–4.5 mIU/L | 1.0–2.0 mIU/L |

***Mental Health Connection:*** TSH is the screening test for thyroid function, but it doesn't tell the whole story. High TSH indicates hypothyroidism (underactive thyroid), which causes fatigue, depression, brain fog, weight gain, and cold intolerance. Low TSH indicates hyperthyroidism (overactive thyroid), which causes anxiety, irritability, insomnia, and racing thoughts. However, TSH can be "normal" while free T3 and T4 are suboptimal. Many people feel best with TSH between 1.0–2.0, even though the reference range goes up to 4.0 or 5.0. Thyroid dysfunction is one of the most common and treatable causes of mental health symptoms.

### Free T4 (Thyroxine)

**What it measures:** The amount of unbound, active thyroid hormone T4 in your blood.

| Test | Reference Range | Functional Range |
|---|---|---|
| Free T4 (Thyroxine) | 0.8–1.8 ng/dL | 1.0–1.5 ng/dL |

*Mental Health Connection:* Free T4 is the storage form of thyroid hormone that gets converted to active T3. Low free T4 contributes to all the symptoms of hypothyroidism: fatigue, depression, difficulty concentrating, and sluggish metabolism. Optimal free T4 is essential for mental clarity and energy, though T3 is the more metabolically active form.

### Free T3 (Triiodothyronine)

**What it measures:** The amount of unbound, active thyroid hormone T3 in your blood—the most metabolically active thyroid hormone.

| Test | Reference Range | Functional Range |
|---|---|---|
| Free T3 (Triiodothyronine) | 2.3–4.2 pg/mL | 3.0–3.8 pg/mL |

*Mental Health Connection:* Free T3 is the hormone that actually does the work at the cellular level. It's critical for energy production, mood regulation, and cognitive function. Low free T3 is one of the most common causes of treatment-resistant depression and chronic fatigue. Your body converts T4 to T3, but this conversion can be impaired by stress, inflammation, nutrient deficiencies (especially selenium and zinc), and certain medications. Many people have "normal" TSH and T4 but low T3, which causes significant symptoms. Optimal T3 is absolutely essential for mental wellness.

## Thyroid Peroxidase Antibodies (TPO)

**What it measures:** Antibodies against an enzyme in your thyroid. Elevated levels indicate autoimmune thyroid disease.

| Test | Reference Range | Functional Range |
|---|---|---|
| Thyroid Peroxidase Antibodies (TPO) | <35 IU/mL | <10 IU/mL |

*Mental Health Connection:* TPO antibodies indicate Hashimoto's thyroiditis, an autoimmune condition where your immune system attacks your thyroid. Even when thyroid hormones are "normal," elevated antibodies indicate ongoing inflammation that can affect brain function. Hashimoto's is strongly associated with depression, anxiety, and cognitive problems—partly due to fluctuating thyroid levels and partly due to the systemic inflammation it causes.

## Reverse T3 (rT3)

**What it measures:** An inactive form of thyroid hormone. Your body produces rT3 by converting T4 into a metabolically inactive mirror image of T3, effectively putting the brakes on metabolism.

| Test | Reference Range | Functional Range |
|---|---|---|
| Reverse T3 (rT3) | 9.2 - 24.1 ng/dL | 9.2-14 ng/dL |

***Mental Health Connection:*** Reverse T3 is the thyroid marker most providers never order and the one that explains why so many women feel terrible despite "normal" thyroid labs. When the body is under chronic stress, caloric restriction, high inflammation, or sleep deprivation, it diverts T4 away from active T3 and toward rT3 as a protective mechanism. The problem is that rT3 competes with T3 for receptor binding but does nothing once it gets there. It's a biological placeholder that blocks the real hormone from doing its job. Elevated rT3 is associated with fatigue, depression, brain fog, weight loss resistance, and cold intolerance, all classic hypothyroid symptoms in a woman whose standard thyroid panel looks clean. The free T3-to-rT3 ratio (free T3 in pg/mL divided by rT3 in ng/dL) is often more clinically useful than any single value. A ratio below 0.2 suggests cellular hypothyroidism even when TSH is within range. This is especially relevant for women in their thirties to fifties dealing with chronic stress, disordered eating history, or perimenopausal transitions.

## Antinuclear Antibodies (ANA)

**What it measures:** Antibodies that target components of cell nuclei. They can indicate autoimmune disease.

| Test | Reference Range | Functional Range |
|---|---|---|
| **Antinuclear Antibodies (ANA)** | Negative | Negative |

***Mental Health Connection:*** Positive ANA indicates possible autoimmune disease, which involves chronic inflammation that affects mental health. Autoimmune conditions are associated with higher rates of depression, anxiety, and cognitive dysfunction due to inflammatory cytokines that cross into the brain.

# 7. Hormone Panel

Hormones are chemical messengers that profoundly influence brain function, mood, energy, and mental health. Sex hormones and stress hormones interact with neurotransmitter systems and can cause symptoms identical to psychiatric disorders when imbalanced. These tests are particularly important for women, as hormonal fluctuations throughout the menstrual cycle, pregnancy, postpartum, and menopause significantly impact mental wellness.

### Cortisol (AM)

**What it measures:** Your primary stress hormone, measured in the morning when it should be at its highest.

| Test | Reference Range | Functional Range |
| --- | --- | --- |
| **Cortisol (AM)** | 6–23 µg/dL | 10–18 µg/dL |

*Mental Health Connection:* Cortisol is your body's main stress hormone and has a natural daily rhythm: high in the morning to help you wake up, low at night to help you sleep. Both high and low cortisol can cause mental health symptoms. High morning cortisol (>20 µg/dL) is associated with chronic stress, anxiety, insomnia, irritability, and difficulty relaxing. It indicates your stress response system is overactive, which eventually leads to burnout. Low morning cortisol (<8 µg/dL) suggests adrenal dysfunction or HPA axis dysregulation; you feel exhausted, can't get out of bed, have low motivation, and struggle to cope with normal stress. This is common after prolonged chronic stress or trauma. Cortisol also affects blood sugar, inflammation, and immune function, all of which impact the brain. Ideally, you want cortisol in the middle of the range: enough to feel energized and able to handle stress, but not so high that you're constantly wired and anxious. A four-point salivary cortisol test (measuring morning, noon, evening, and night) gives a much better picture of your daily rhythm than a single blood draw.

## DHEA-S

**What it measures:** A hormone produced by your adrenal glands that serves as a precursor to sex hormones and has independent effects on mood and energy.

| Test | Reference Range | Functional Range |
|---|---|---|
| **DHEA-S** | 35–430 μg/dL (F), 80–560 μg/dL (M) | 200–350 μg/dL (F), 350–500 μg/dL (M) |

*Mental Health Connection:* DHEA-S is often called the "anti-stress" or "youth" hormone because it has neuroprotective effects and typically declines with age and chronic stress. It balances the effects of cortisol; while cortisol breaks things down under stress, DHEA helps build things back up. Low DHEA-S is associated with depression, fatigue, low motivation, poor stress resilience, and cognitive decline. It's particularly important for recovery from chronic stress or burnout. DHEA supports brain function by promoting neuroplasticity, protecting against inflammation, and supporting neurotransmitter production. The cortisol-to-DHEA ratio is important; high cortisol with low DHEA suggests burnout and impaired stress resilience. DHEA levels naturally decline with age, so what's "normal" for a sixty-year-old is much lower than for a thirty-year-old. Low DHEA in younger people often indicates chronic stress, overtraining, or adrenal dysfunction. Supplementing DHEA (under medical supervision) can improve mood and energy in people with documented low levels, though it's important to monitor, as it converts to other hormones.

## Testosterone, Total — Female

**What it measures:** The total amount of testosterone in the blood. Women produce much less testosterone than men, but it's still essential for mental health.

| Test | Reference Range | Functional Range |
| --- | --- | --- |
| **Testosterone, Total — Female** | 15–70 ng/dL | 30–60 ng/dL |

***Mental Health Connection:*** Testosterone isn't just a "male" hormone. Women need it too for motivation, confidence, libido, energy, and mood stability. Low testosterone in women causes fatigue, depression, low motivation, difficulty building muscle, decreased libido, and brain fog. It's particularly common after childbirth, during perimenopause/menopause, with birth control use, and in women with PCOS. Testosterone supports dopamine function, which is critical for motivation, pleasure, and focus. Very low testosterone (<20 ng/dL) can feel like treatment-resistant depression. Many women with testosterone in the 15–25 ng/dL range experience significant improvements in mood, energy, and mental clarity when levels are optimized to 40–50 ng/dL. High testosterone in women (>70 ng/dL) can indicate PCOS and is associated with anxiety, irritability, and mood swings due to its conversion to estrogen and its effects on other hormones.

## Testosterone, Total — Male

**What it measures:** The total amount of testosterone in the blood, essential for male physical and mental health.

| Test | Reference Range | Functional Range |
|---|---|---|
| **Testosterone, Total — Male** | 264–916 ng/dL | 500–800 ng/dL |

***Mental Health Connection:*** Testosterone is critical for male mental health, affecting mood, motivation, confidence, energy, and cognitive function. Low testosterone (<300 ng/dL) causes depression, fatigue, low motivation, irritability, brain fog, decreased libido, and difficulty building muscle. It's increasingly common due to obesity, stress, poor sleep, and environmental factors. Low testosterone impairs dopamine function, leading to anhedonia (inability to experience pleasure) and lack of drive. Many men with "treatment-resistant depression" actually have low testosterone. Testosterone levels naturally decline with age, but significant symptoms shouldn't be dismissed as "just aging." Men with testosterone in the 300–400 ng/dL range (technically "normal") often experience significant improvements in mood, energy, and mental clarity when optimized to 600–700 ng/dL. Very high testosterone (>900 ng/dL) can cause irritability, aggression, and mood swings, though this is less common unless using exogenous testosterone. Testosterone should be measured in the morning when levels are highest.

### Estradiol (E2)

**What it measures:** The primary and most potent form of estrogen, which has powerful effects on brain function and mood.

| Test | Reference Range | Functional Range |
| --- | --- | --- |
| **Estradiol (E2)** | Varies by cycle | Follicular: 50–80 pg/mL, Luteal: 80–150 pg/mL |

*Mental Health Connection:* Estradiol profoundly affects brain function, mood, and cognition. It supports serotonin production, protects neurons, reduces inflammation, and promotes neuroplasticity. Low estradiol causes depression, anxiety, brain fog, memory problems, insomnia, and hot flashes. This is particularly common during perimenopause, postpartum, and with birth control that suppresses estrogen. Many women experience dramatic mood changes with estrogen fluctuations; PMS, PMDD, postpartum depression, and perimenopausal depression are all influenced by estradiol levels and fluctuations. Estradiol enhances the effects of serotonin, so low estrogen can look identical to depression. High estradiol (>200 pg/mL in the luteal phase) can cause anxiety, irritability, breast tenderness, and mood swings; this is "estrogen dominance" and is often due to low progesterone relative to estrogen. Estradiol must be interpreted in the context of the menstrual cycle phase and in relation to progesterone. For women on birth control, levels may be suppressed, which can contribute to mood issues. For postmenopausal women, estradiol is naturally low. Hormone replacement therapy can significantly improve mood and cognition in some women.

## Progesterone

**What it measures:** A hormone produced primarily in the second half of the menstrual cycle (luteal phase) that has calming, antianxiety effects.

| Test | Reference Range | Functional Range |
|---|---|---|
| **Progesterone** | <1.0 ng/mL (follicular), 5–20 ng/mL (luteal) | 10–25 ng/mL (luteal) |

***Mental Health Connection:*** Progesterone is the "calming" hormone with powerful antianxiety effects. It's converted in the brain to allopregnanolone, which enhances GABA function—your brain's primary calming neurotransmitter. Low progesterone in the luteal phase causes anxiety, insomnia, irritability, racing thoughts, and PMS/PMDD symptoms. It's extremely common in women with irregular cycles, chronic stress, PCOS, and perimenopause. Low progesterone relative to estrogen ("estrogen dominance") causes mood swings, anxiety, breast tenderness, and heavy periods. Progesterone also supports thyroid function and protects against estrogen's proliferative effects. Many women with anxiety and insomnia have undiagnosed low progesterone. Progesterone should be measured in the luteal phase (day twenty-one of a twenty-eight–day cycle, or seven days after ovulation) because it's naturally low in the follicular phase. Levels below 10 ng/mL in the luteal phase suggest inadequate progesterone production, which significantly impacts mood and sleep. Very low progesterone can also indicate anovulatory cycles (not ovulating), which is common with stress and PCOS. Bioidentical progesterone supplementation can be life-changing for women with documented low levels, particularly for anxiety and sleep issues.

# 8. Urinalysis

Urinalysis examines the physical, chemical, and microscopic properties of urine. While primarily used to detect urinary and kidney disorders, several components can affect overall health and mental well-being.

### Specific Gravity

**What it measures:** Measures the concentration of your urine, indicating hydration status.

| Test | Reference Range | Functional Range |
| --- | --- | --- |
| **Specific Gravity** | 1.005–1.030 | 1.010–1.020 |

***Mental Health Connection:*** Specific gravity reflects hydration. Dehydration (high specific gravity) impairs cognitive function, causes fatigue, and worsens mood. Even mild dehydration can significantly affect mental performance and increase anxiety. Adequate hydration is essential for optimal brain function.

### pH

**What it measures:** The acidity or alkalinity of your urine.

| Test | Reference Range | Functional Range |
| --- | --- | --- |
| **pH** | 4.5–8.0 | 6.0–7.0 |

***Mental Health Connection:*** Urine pH reflects your body's acid-base balance and metabolic processes. Consistently very acidic or alkaline urine can indicate dietary imbalances or metabolic issues. While not directly tied to mental health, pH abnormalities can reflect poor diet or metabolic dysfunction that affects overall health.

## Protein

**What it measures:** Detects protein in urine, which normally shouldn't be there.

| Test | Reference Range | Functional Range |
| --- | --- | --- |
| **Protein** | Negative | Negative |

*Mental Health Connection:* Protein in urine indicates kidney damage or dysfunction. When kidneys aren't working properly, toxins accumulate that affect brain function, causing confusion, fatigue, and mood changes.

## Glucose

**What it measures:** Detects glucose in urine. Normally glucose is reabsorbed by the kidneys.

| Test | Reference Range | Functional Range |
| --- | --- | --- |
| **Glucose** | Negative | Negative |

*Mental Health Connection:* Glucose in urine indicates very high blood sugar (typically >180 mg/dL), suggesting diabetes or severe hyperglycemia. Chronically elevated blood sugar damages blood vessels and nerves throughout the body, including in the brain, leading to cognitive decline and mood disorders.

## Ketones

**What it measures:** Detects ketones, which are produced when your body burns fat for fuel instead of glucose.

| Test | Reference Range | Functional Range |
| --- | --- | --- |
| **Ketones** | Negative | Negative (or trace if fasting) |

*Mental Health Connection:* Ketones in urine can indicate diabetic ketoacidosis (a medical emergency), starvation, or intentional ketogenic dieting. While nutritional ketosis can have benefits for some people with mood disorders and epilepsy, high ketone levels without proper context can indicate metabolic crisis.

## Blood

**What it measures:** Detects blood in urine, which can indicate infection, kidney stones, or other issues.

| Test | Reference Range | Functional Range |
| --- | --- | --- |
| **Blood** | Negative | Negative |

*Mental Health Connection:* Blood in urine requires investigation for the underlying cause. Chronic infections or kidney problems can contribute to systemic inflammation and fatigue that affect mental health.

## Leukocyte Esterase

**What it measures:** Detects white blood cells in urine, indicating infection or inflammation.

| Test | Reference Range | Functional Range |
| --- | --- | --- |
| **Leukocyte Esterase** | Negative | Negative |

***Mental Health Connection:*** Positive leukocyte esterase suggests urinary tract infection, which can cause confusion, agitation, and mood changes, especially in older adults. Treating infections is important for maintaining mental clarity.

## Nitrites

**What it measures:** Detects bacteria in urine that convert nitrates to nitrites.

| Test | Reference Range | Functional Range |
| --- | --- | --- |
| **Nitrites** | Negative | Negative |

***Mental Health Connection:*** Positive nitrites indicate bacterial urinary tract infection. UTIs can cause systemic symptoms including confusion, irritability, and fatigue that affect mental state.

**How to Use This Lab Tracker**

This lab tracker is meant to empower you to understand your lab results and have informed conversations with your healthcare provider. Here's how to make the most of it:

1. Request copies of your lab results from your doctor. You have a right to your medical records.
2. Compare your values to both the reference range and the functional range provided here.
3. Pay special attention to values that are "normal" but not optimal; these often contribute to symptoms.
4. Read the mental health connections for any tests that are out of the functional range.
5. Bring this information to your doctor to discuss potential interventions.
6. Remember that lab values are just one piece of the puzzle. How you feel matters more than any number.

*Your health journey is unique to you. Use this guide as a starting point for conversations with healthcare providers who understand that optimal health requires more than just "normal" lab values. You deserve to feel your best.*

# COMPREHENSIVE GLOSSARY

*A detailed, plain-English reference with just enough attitude to keep you awake.*

## NEUROCHEMISTRY AND NEUROTRANSMITTERS

**Acetate, Propionate, Butyrate (SCFAs):** Short-chain fatty acids from fiber-fed microbes that influence inflammation, gut integrity, and brain signaling.

**Acetylcholine (ACh):** Neurotransmitter for learning, attention, and muscle activation. Think memory plus mind–body coordination.

**Adenosine:** Sleep pressure molecule. Builds up while you are awake; caffeine sits on its receptors and fakes alertness.

**Arachidonic Acid Eicosanoids:** Inflammation-signaling molecules. Balanced by EPA-derived eicosanoids.

**Brain-Derived Neurotrophic Factor (BDNF):** Fertilizer for neurons, supports plasticity, learning, and mood.

**Dopamine:** Motivation and reward signaling. Peaks with progress and novelty, crashes with chaos and no wins.

**Endocannabinoids (Anandamide, 2-AG):** Your internal "runner's high" messengers. Mood smoothing, pain blunting.

**Endorphins:** Body-made opioids that dull pain and lift mood, often after effort or laughter.

**GABA (Gamma-Aminobutyric Acid):** Primary calming neurotransmitter. Helps stop spirals and supports sleep.

**Glutamate:** Primary excitatory neurotransmitter. Great for learning, not great when chronically elevated.

**Norepinephrine (Noradrenaline):** Alerting chemical for focus and vigilance. Too much equals jittery mind.

**Oxytocin:** Connection and trust hormone, also modulates stress reactivity.

**Serotonin:** Mood stabilizer involved in appetite, sleep, digestion, and contentment.

**Tryptophan:** Amino acid precursor to serotonin. Needs iron, B6, and magnesium to convert efficiently.

**Tyrosine:** Amino acid precursor to dopamine and norepinephrine.

## BRAIN, NERVES, AND NETWORKS

**Amygdala:** Alarm system for threat detection. Sometimes dramatic.

**Anterior Cingulate Cortex (ACC):** Error detection and emotional regulation hub.

**Default Mode Network (DMN, Automatic Thought Network):** Self-talk and mind-wandering network. Overactive DMN correlates with rumination.

**Enteric Nervous System (ENS):** "Second brain" in the gut. Runs digestion and talks to the head office.

**Glymphatic System:** Brain's waste-clearance system, most active during deep sleep and supported by regular movement.

**Hippocampus:** Memory consolidation center. Sensitive to stress, loves BDNF.

**HPA Axis (Hypothalamic-Pituitary-Adrenal):** Stress command chain that sets cortisol rhythms.

**Neuroinflammation:** Immune activation inside the brain that alters mood and cognition.

**Neuroplasticity:** Brain's ability to rewire. Practice and repetition reshape circuits.

**Vagus Nerve:** Bidirectional superhighway between brain and organs. Breathwork, humming, and cold exposure can raise vagal tone.

## HORMONES AND RELATED CHEMISTRY

**Adiponectin:** Hormone from fat cells that improves insulin sensitivity.

**Cortisol:** Stress hormone that follows a diurnal curve. Chronic elevation disrupts sleep, mood, and metabolism.

**COMT, MAO:** Enzymes that clear catecholamines. Genetic variants change how quickly you metabolize stress chemicals.

**DHEA:** Adrenal hormone that counters some cortisol effects and supports resilience.

**Estrogen (Estradiol, E2):** Influences serotonin, dopamine, and synaptic plasticity. Fluctuations affect mood.

**Ghrelin:** Appetite signal from the stomach that rises before meals.

**Hepcidin:** Regulates iron absorption. Chronically high hepcidin blocks iron uptake.

**Insulin:** Hormone that ushers glucose into cells. High levels over time blunt sensitivity and strain the brain.

**Leptin:** Satiety signal from fat tissue. Resistance equals constant hunger.

**Progesterone:** Calming, GABA-supportive hormone. Drops pre-menses can worsen anxiety.

**Prolactin:** Hormone for lactation. Elevated levels can affect mood and cycles.

**Testosterone:** Motivation, drive, and energy. Excessively low levels can reduce mood and focus.

**Thyroid Hormones (T4, T3):** Metabolic pace setters. Low thyroid function mimics depression and brain fog.

**Thyroid Stimulating Hormone (TSH):** Pituitary signal to the thyroid. High TSH often indicates low thyroid output.

## METABOLIC HEALTH, GLUCOSE, AND ENERGY

**Adenosine Triphosphate (ATP):** Cellular energy currency.

**Beta-Oxidation:** Process of turning fats into energy in mitochondria.

**Gluconeogenesis:** Making glucose from non-carb sources during long gaps between meals or intense exercise.

**GLUT4:** Transporter that moves glucose into muscle after exercise.

**Glycemic Variability:** Size of blood sugar swings. Lower variability equals steadier mood and cognition.

**HbA1c:** Three-month average of blood glucose. Lower is generally better within normal range.

**HOMA-IR:** Insulin-resistance index calculated from fasting glucose and insulin.

**Mitochondria:** Power plants of the cell. Sensitive to nutrients, toxins, and movement.

**Reactive Hypoglycemia:** Post-meal sugar crash that triggers adrenaline and anxiety.

**VO2 Max:** Capacity to use oxygen during exercise, a marker of cardiorespiratory fitness.

## LIPIDS AND OMEGA-3S

**Alpha-Linolenic Acid (ALA):** Plant omega-3 that converts poorly to EPA and DHA.

**Eicosapentaenoic Acid (EPA):** Anti-inflammatory omega-3 that supports mood and immune signaling.

**Docosahexaenoic Acid (DHA):** Structural omega-3 that keeps neuronal membranes fluid.

**Omega-6-to-Omega-3 Ratio:** Balance of dietary fats. Lower ratios are generally less inflammatory.

**Triglyceride Form vs. Ethyl Ester:** Supplement forms of omega-3s. Triglyceride or re-esterified triglyceride tends to absorb better.

## VITAMINS, MINERALS, AND COFACTORS

**B1 (Thiamine):** Carbohydrate metabolism and nerve function.

**B2 (Riboflavin):** Mitochondrial energy, also a cofactor for MTHFR.

**B3 (Niacin):** Builds NAD, central to cellular energy.

**B5 (Pantothenic Acid):** Coenzyme A production, stress hormone synthesis.

**B6 (Pyridoxine, P5P):** Cofactor for serotonin, dopamine, and GABA production.

**B9 (Folate, Methylfolate):** Methyl donor for neurotransmitter and DNA synthesis. Folate is food form; folic acid is synthetic.

**B12 (Cobalamin, Methylcobalamin):** Nerve integrity and red blood cell production. Low B12 equals fatigue and brain fog.

**Choline (Citicoline, Alpha-GPC):** Precursor to acetylcholine and phospholipids, supports attention and memory.

**Creatine:** Recycles cellular energy, helpful for brain performance under stress or sleep loss.

**Ferritin:** Iron storage protein. Low ferritin often equals low iron reserves.

**Iodine:** Required for thyroid hormone synthesis.

**Iron:** Required for dopamine synthesis and oxygen delivery. Deficiency causes fatigue and restless legs.

**Magnesium (Glycinate, Citrate, Threonate):** Calms nerves, supports sleep, and participates in hundreds of reactions.

**Selenium:** Needed for thyroid hormone activation and antioxidant enzymes.

**Transferrin Saturation, TIBC:** Iron transport metrics used with ferritin to evaluate status.

**Vitamin C:** Antioxidant and collagen cofactor. Helps recycle other antioxidants.

**Vitamin D3 (Cholecalciferol):** Hormone-like vitamin that modulates immunity, mood, and calcium balance.

**Vitamin E (Tocopherols, Tocotrienols):** Lipid-phase antioxidant protecting membranes.

**Vitamin K2 (MK-7):** Directs calcium to bones and away from arteries.

**Zinc:** Cofactor for neurotransmitters and immune function. Too much blocks copper and iron.

## GUT, MICROBIOME, AND DIGESTION

**Dysbiosis:** Unbalanced gut ecosystem linked to mood and immune issues.

**Fermented Foods:** Foods with live cultures, e.g., yogurt, kefir, kimchi, sauerkraut.

**Histamine Intolerance:** Reduced breakdown of histamine—causing headaches, hives, and anxiety after certain foods.

**Intestinal Permeability:** Loosening of gut tight junctions that lets immune-provoking molecules into the bloodstream.

***Lactobacillus, Bifidobacterium:*** Common beneficial genera that produce GABA, SCFAs, and vitamins.

**Lipopolysaccharide (LPS):** Bacterial fragment that can drive inflammation if it escapes the gut.

**Mast Cells:** Immune cells in gut and brain that release histamine and cytokines.

**Microbiota-Gut-Brain Axis:** Communication between microbes and the nervous system via neural, immune, and endocrine routes.

**Motility, Migrating Motor Complex (MMC):** Cyclical waves that sweep the small intestine between meals. Help prevent bacterial overgrowth.

**Prebiotics:** Fibers that feed good microbes, e.g., inulin, FOS, GOS, resistant starch.

**Probiotics:** Live microbes that confer a benefit when consumed in adequate amounts.

**Psychobiotics:** Probiotic strains with evidence for mood or stress support.

**Short-Chain Fatty Acids (SCFAs):** Microbial metabolites that maintain gut barrier and regulate inflammation.

## IMMUNITY, INFLAMMATION, AND OXIDATIVE STRESS

**Cytokines (IL-6, TNF-α, IL-1β):** Immune messengers. Chronic elevation correlates with low mood and brain fog.

**C-Reactive Protein (CRP, hs-CRP):** Blood marker of systemic inflammation.

**Glutathione (GSH):** Master antioxidant. Depleted by stress, toxins, and illness.

**Mast Cell Activation:** Hypersensitive mast cells releasing histamine and cytokines.

**Microglia:** Brain immune cells that prune synapses and, when overactivated, drive neuroinflammation.

**NRF2:** Transcription factor that turns on antioxidant defense genes.

**Oxidative Stress:** Imbalance between free radicals and antioxidants that damages lipids, proteins, and DNA.

**ROS, RNS:** Reactive oxygen and nitrogen species that, in excess, harm cells.

**SOD, Catalase, Glutathione Peroxidase:** Core antioxidant enzymes.

## MOVEMENT, EXERCISE, AND PHYSIOLOGY

**Afterburn (EPOC):** Elevated oxygen use and calorie burn after intense exercise.

**BDNF Response to Exercise:** Movement increases BDNF and supports learning and mood.

**High-Intensity Interval Training (HIIT):** Short intervals of hard effort with recovery. Efficient but not required.

**Heart Rate Variability (HRV):** Variation between heartbeats. Higher HRV usually means better stress resilience.

**Irisin and Myokines:** Muscle-released signaling proteins that influence brain and metabolism.

**Lactate:** Metabolite that can be shuttled as fuel. Not just a waste product.

**Non-Exercise Activity Thermogenesis (NEAT):** All the movement that is not a workout, for example walking, fidgeting, stairs.

**Progressive Overload:** Gradual increase in training stress that drives adaptation.

**Resistance Training:** Strength work using body weight or external load to build muscle and insulin sensitivity.

**Zone 2 Training:** Conversational-pace cardio that builds mitochondria and fat oxidation.

## MINDFULNESS, PSYCHOLOGY, AND SLEEP

**Allostatic Load:** Total wear and tear from repeated stress responses.

**Attentional Control:** Ability to select and sustain focus.

**Circadian Rhythm:** Twenty-four-hour internal clock set by light and behavior. Morning light anchors it.

**Cognitive Reappraisal:** Reframing thoughts to change emotional impact.

**DMN Quieting:** Practices that reduce mind wandering and rumination, e.g., breathwork and meditation.

**Interoception:** Sensing internal body signals like heartbeat and breath.

**Melatonin:** Darkness signal that primes sleep onset. Blue light late at night suppresses it.

**Metacognition:** Observing your own thinking, helpful for stepping out of loops.

**Parasympathetic Activation:** Rest-and-digest mode that slows heart rate and aids digestion.

**Sympathetic Activation:** Fight-or-flight mode for fast responses.

**Sleep Architecture:** Stages and cycles across a night. Deep sleep favors brain cleanup; REM favors memory integration.

**Slow-Wave Sleep:** Deep, restorative sleep tied to glymphatic clearance and growth-hormone release.

## GENETICS AND METHYLATION

**5-HTTLPR:** Serotonin transporter gene variant linked to stress sensitivity.

**COMT Val158Met:** Variant that slows catecholamine breakdown. It can heighten sensitivity to stress or stimulants.

**Homocysteine:** Sulfur-containing metabolite. Elevated levels signal methylation issues and vascular risk.

**Methylation:** Biochemical tagging process required for neurotransmitters, DNA repair, and detox.

**MAOA, MAOB:** Enzymes that degrade monoamines like serotonin and dopamine.

**Methylmalonic Acid (MMA):** Functional marker of B12 status. High MMA suggests low B12 activity.

**MTHFR:** Gene that helps process folate. Variants can raise homocysteine and change folate needs.

## LABS, PANELS, AND RANGES

**25-Hydroxyvitamin D [25(OH)D]:** Storage form used to gauge vitamin D status.

**Complete Blood Count (CBC):** Red and white cells and platelets. Screens for anemia and infection.

**Comprehensive Metabolic Panel (CMP):** Electrolytes, kidney and liver function, glucose.

**Cortisol a.m./p.m.:** Diurnal pattern check. A healthy curve peaks in the morning and declines through the day.

**Estradiol, Progesterone, Testosterone:** Key sex hormones. Timing in the cycle matters for interpretation.

**Fasting Glucose:** Morning sugar level after no food. Often best between about 75 and 85 mg/dL for brain steadiness.

**Fasting Insulin:** Helps estimate insulin resistance when paired with glucose. Often best under about 5 μIU/mL.

**Ferritin, Iron, TIBC, Transferrin Sat:** Iron panel components.

**HbA1c:** Average glucose over about three months. Lower normal values are typically brain friendlier.

**hs-CRP:** High-sensitivity CRP for subtle inflammation.

**Lipid Panel:** Cholesterol fractions and triglycerides. HDL is generally protective; LDL needs context.

**LFTs (ALT, AST, ALP, Bilirubin):** Liver enzymes and bile markers.

**Oral Glucose Tolerance Test (OGTT):** Measures response to a glucose load.

**Thyroid Panel (TSH, Free T4, Free T3, rT3):** Measures thyroid function and conversion.

## FOODS, PATTERNS, AND DIETARY TERMS

**Electrolytes:** Sodium, potassium, magnesium, calcium. Keep nerves firing and muscles contracting.

**Glycemic Load:** A measure of how a food impacts blood sugar considering portion size.

**Mediterranean Pattern:** Vegetables, legumes, whole grains, olive oil, nuts, fish. Anti-inflammatory and microbiome friendly.

**Polyphenols:** Plant defense compounds that act as signaling molecules and antioxidants in humans.

**Resistant Starch:** Starch that resists digestion, feeds microbes, and raises butyrate.

**Ultra-Processed Foods (UPFs):** Industrial formulations that spike glucose, dopamine, and cravings while skimping on nutrients.

## SUPPLEMENTS, BOTANICALS, AND "SMART" COMPOUNDS

**Ashwagandha *(Withania somnifera)*:** Adaptogen that may lower perceived stress and support sleep.

**Citicoline, Alpha-GPC:** Choline sources for acetylcholine and membrane support.

**Creatine Monohydrate:** Brain and muscle energy buffer, especially helpful when sleep deprived or plant-based.

**Fish Oil, Algae Oil:** Sources of EPA and DHA. Check actual EPA and DHA dose per serving.

**Holy Basil, Tulsi:** Herb with traditional use for mood and glycemic balance.

**Lion's Mane *(Hericium erinaceus)*:** Mushroom with preliminary data for nerve growth support.

**L-Theanine:** Tea amino acid that smooths caffeine and promotes relaxed focus.

**Magnesium Glycinate:** Gentle form for calm and sleep.

**Magnesium Threonate:** Form that may cross the blood–brain barrier more effectively.

**Methylcobalamin, Methylfolate:** Activated forms of B12 and B9 for those with methylation issues.

**N-Acetylcysteine (NAC):** Precursor to glutathione. Studied for mood and compulsive behaviors.

**Reishi** *(Ganoderma lucidum):* Mushroom used for immune modulation and calm.

**Resveratrol:** Polyphenol that activates antioxidant defenses.

*Rhodiola rosea:* Adaptogen for fatigue and focus, useful in high-demand phases.

## DEVICES, METRICS, AND METHODS

**Actigraphy:** Wearable movement tracking that estimates sleep and activity.

**Continuous Glucose Monitor (CGM):** Sensor that tracks glucose patterns in real time.

**Exposure Protocols:** Gradual, controlled encounters with triggers to retrain the threat response.

**Incremental Breathwork:** Short, structured breathing sets to raise vagal tone.

**Rate of Perceived Exertion (RPE):** Self-rated intensity scale for workouts.

## UNITS, ABBREVIATIONS, AND CONVERSIONS

**mg/dL:** Milligrams per deciliter, common for glucose and lipids.

**ng/mL:** Nanograms per milliliter, common for vitamin D and hormones.

**μIU/mL:** Micro-international units per milliliter, common for insulin and TSH.

**IU:** International unit, potency measure for vitamins like D.

**mcg, μg:** Microgram; 1,000 micrograms equals 1 milligram.

## QUICK REFERENCE MINI-MAPS

**Calm Inflammation:** Omega-3s, polyphenols, fiber, sleep, movement, stress skills, diverse microbes.

**Make Dopamine:** Tyrosine, iron, B6, folate, B12, creatine, sleep, progress on tiny goals.

**Make Serotonin:** Tryptophan, B6, iron, magnesium, sunlight, steady glucose, calm gut.

**Steady Glucose:** Protein plus fiber plus healthy fat, movement after meals, fewer liquid sugars, adequate sleep.

www.ingramcontent.com/pod-product-compliance
Lightning Source LLC
Chambersburg PA
CBHW051227050726
47594CB00001B/63